FITNESS CONFIDENTIAL

by

Vinnie Tortorich
&
Dean Lorey

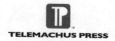

TELEMACHUS PRESS

Although this book is non-fiction, certain names have been changed.

Cover designed by Patrick Bradley

Interior photos taken by:
Weight Room by Cy Tortorich
Shirtless, white shorts by Michael Tortorich
Serena and Dean by Vinnie Tortorich
Group shot by Marie Tortorich
Vinnie on bike, Rainbow, Vinnie with milkshake, Vinnie on long desert road, Vinnie shirtless by Serena Scott Thomas
Hug by Chris Kostman

Cover photo:
Copyright © David Zaugh

Published by Telemachus Press, LLC
http://www.telemachuspress.com

Visit the authors' websites:
http://www.vinnietortorich.com
http://www.deanlorey.com

ISBN: 978-1-939337-91-7 (eBook)
ISBN: 978-1-939337-92-4 (Paperback)

Version 2013.06.20

Printed in the United States of America

10 9 8 7 6 5 4 3 2 1

FITNESS CONFIDENTIAL

Chapter One
I'M YOUR TRAINER

"WE UNDERSTAND YOU'RE the go-to guy for taking weight off people."

I was sitting in a conference room, staring at a rogue's gallery of Hollywood types. There was a top showrunner preparing a new sitcom, the managers of the show's star, plus an exec from Disney along with the usual group of faceless nobodies who seem to be in every meeting in Tinseltown filling up space.

I wasn't exactly sure how to respond. It was the early nineties. I'd only been in L.A. a couple of years and my personal training career was just starting to gain traction.

"Yeah, I'm the guy," I said, wondering how they even got my name.

They glanced at each other nervously. It was clear they had a problem, or at least they thought they did, and somehow I was supposed to solve it.

"Can you take thirty-five pounds off someone?" the manager asked.

"That depends," I replied. "Does this person have thirty-five pounds to lose?"

Again, they glanced at each other. Finally, the network exec spoke. "We think so."

"Then, yeah," I said. "Sure."

There was a visible sigh of relief. The showrunner leaned toward me. "Can you do it in six weeks?"

More than five pounds a week. That's a tall order. Not to mention unhealthy, which is what I told them.

The manager stared at me, then wrote something on a slip of paper. He slid it over to me.

It said: $10,000.

I stared at it for a minute. I've never been a money guy, but I'm not crazy.

"Yeah, no problem," I said. I figured I could help whoever this was take at least twenty, twenty-five pounds off in a healthy way and everyone would be satisfied. Which raised a larger question.

"Exactly who are we talking about here?" I asked. The whole thing was so shrouded in secrecy I was wondering if they were bringing in the First Lady to do a sitcom.

The network executive narrowed his eyes. "You know who Lucille Ball is?"

"Yeah," I replied. "But it's gonna be hard to train a dead person."

"We're creating the new Lucille Ball. She's going to star in a sitcom for us." He said her name. You'd recognize it. "She's talented, but she failed her screen test. The issue is the weight. Your job is to make that issue go away."

It was like being in *The Godfather,* except I was the only Italian in the room.

"No problem," I said. "I'll get to work."

Believe it or not, this was a typical day for me. I never knew what to expect when I went to work in the morning. One time I got a phone call from a Beverly Hills housewife who told me she needed my help to get into shape. I showed up to find her in a silk robe. She stripped it off to reveal a smoking-hot body.

"I want you to make this better," she said. "I want a body like a porn star."

I didn't have the heart to tell her she was already there. Who's going to deny a woman willing to strip naked on the first workout?

Then there was the male film star who hired me, paid me three times to show up, then fired me without ever meeting me. His reasoning? He wasn't feeling my "vibe." I told him he might be able to feel it better if we were ever actually in the same room.

One of the best moments was the first time I heard my name mentioned on *The Tonight Show*. That was when I felt I'd arrived.

I've been a Beverly Hills personal trainer for over twenty-two years and I've seen it all. Along the way, I've helped hundreds of people get into shape. CEOs, celebrities, athletes—you name it. Whenever I meet people, the first thing they usually tell me is what went into their mouth and came out their ass. They're looking for my blessing or forgiveness, like I'm a priest of fat. The truth is, I like hearing about it—but I'm the only one. You want to know who doesn't care what diet you're on?

Everyone else.

But I care.

And I've been caring a long time. In the past quarter century, I've learned all the dirt there is about the fitness game—and even created some of it. I know where the bodies are buried. And I'm going to show them to you.

I'm going to expose the nasty little tricks health clubs play to get you to sign up. These guys make used car salesmen look like they belong in a nunnery. Note to nuns: I'm coming after you, too. But don't worry, not only will I show you how to get the best deal, I'll show you how to use the place to your advantage once you're in.

I'm going to tell you how you can figure out which personal trainers are great and which ones suck. I have a degree in fitness from Tulane University along with the pre-requisite muscles and bright teeth. Most of the other trainers only have two of those three.

I'm going to tell you which so-called "fitness products" are worth your cash and which ones aren't worth the box they came in.

I'm looking at you, Thighmaster.

I'll tell you everything. And, along the way, I'm going to piss a lot of people off. They don't call me "America's Angriest Trainer" for nothing.

Over the years, I've noticed that most people don't take my career seriously. A doctor once called me a "fringe player" because he couldn't understand what I was doing with my life.

"You're way too smart to be a trainer," he told me.

You'd be surprised how much I get that attitude.

When I was a kid, the job didn't even exist. All my friends wanted to drive a fire truck when they grew up, but I never heard any of them say, "Hey, I think I want to be a trainer."

I guess I understand that. My life isn't exactly what you'd call normal. If there's a white picket fence around, I've never walked through it.

I don't draw a weekly paycheck. In fact, the work is all free-lance. I only get paid when I show up at a client's door and they hand me a check.

I don't work nine to five. I wake up at 4 a.m. to get ready to meet my first client at six. People ask me why I need two hours and I tell them "one of us has to be awake and I'm the one getting paid." Usually, I don't have my last client until after 10 p.m. I work when my client is free.

When most people are off on the weekends, I'm going into my busy period. In fact, the very concept of a "week" has no meaning for me. When I'm driving around to meet my clients, I hear guys on the radio talking about "Blue Monday," and how Wednesday is "hump day," and how it's time to celebrate "TGIF."

It's all the same to me.

Saturday night is the only night that's a little different, because I'll usually pour myself a glass of scotch—but only one. Remember, I have to meet my first client at 6 a.m. the next morning. On Sunday.

I live in my car. Not really, but it feels that way. I work a minimum of sixteen-hour days and at least four of those are spent on the freeways in L.A. When asked what I do for a living, I usually answer, "I drive!"

The only meal I eat at home is breakfast. Lunch could be at ten in the morning or four in the afternoon, depending on my client's schedule. Dinner, if I can get it, is whenever I can squeeze it in.

I spend my day getting people to do things they don't want to do. Lift heavy weights, run long distances, cycle up mountains. I'm half drill sergeant; half armchair psychologist and I have to be as enthusiastic with the first client as with the last. They don't want to know you've had a rough day—they've had a rough day.

When I step foot into my client's homes, I usually feel like the help. I'm just another person they employ, but instead of fixing their cars or appliances, I'm fixing them. The only difference between the rest of the help and me is that I see them at their most vulnerable.

And, because of that, I hear everything.

Why do women go to hairdressers just to get their hair blown out? They could just as easily do that at home for free, but they'll spend the time and effort to drive all the way to a hair salon just so that they can gossip about their lives to a friendly ear.

Same with personal trainers.

Unlike at a hair salon where there's no privacy, the client and I are alone at the client's house, talking about extremely personal things. It's not uncommon for a woman to strip down naked in front of me to show me a place that hurts or an area they want to improve. I've had women ask me to check their breasts for lumps. I explain to them that I'm not a doctor and wouldn't know what a lump is supposed to feel like, but they're comfortable with me and want me to check anyway.

I always do … and then recommend that they see a doctor.

Speaking of breasts, Beverly Hills is the fake tit capital of the world. I can't begin to tell you the amount of clients I've had that get a boob job and, as soon as they see me, pop open their tops, eager to show off their new purchase. They all ask the same question.

"Do these look real?"

I always give them the same answer.

"Yes."

That reminds me of a Vinnie-ism.

If you want me to tell you the truth, I'm going to have to lie.

Truth is, I've yet to see a boob job I liked. But I sure have massaged a lot of them. Every time I hear that a client is going to get a boob job, I immediately wonder when this uncomfortable conversation is going to take place.

Them: "This may sound kind of strange—"

As soon as I hear "this may sound kind of strange" I know I'm about to be asked to do what I call the "jug rub."

Them: "This may sound kind of strange but my doctor says, in order to avoid building up scar tissue—which would make my boobs feel unnatural—they have to be massaged several times a day." I usually pretend that this is the first time I've ever heard this.

Me: "Oh, really?"

Them: "Would you mind? Is it weird for me to ask you to massage them?"

Me: "Can't you get your husband to do that?"

They usually answer one of two ways.

Them: "He always says he's too tired."

OR

Them: "As soon as he starts to play with them, we end up having sex."

Whenever I hear that, I always wonder why she thinks that, when *I'm* playing with them, *I'm* not going to want to have sex. Amazingly, I've never once let the situation get inappropriate—aside from how inappropriate the whole thing is.

And it's not just the women.

No, I've never massaged a guy's breasts, but I do have one client who likes to take the occasional session to have me shave his back because his wife refuses to do it. No problem. I'm handy with a razor. And to take the sting out of the awkwardness of the whole deal, while I'm doing it, we usually talk football—even when it's not football season.

Many women think the only thing guys care about are their penises. I've got news for these ladies. They're right. The top three questions I get from guys all deal with their schlongs.

Them: "Hey, we're about the same age, right?"

This is the male version of the female conversation starter "this may sound kind of strange." As soon as a guy says to me, "Hey, we're about the same age, right?" I know that one of three questions is about to be asked.

QUESTION ONE

Them: "Hey, we're about the same age, right?"

Me (dreading this): "Yeah."

Them: "Your thing ever go limp when you're having sex?"

Me: "Uh ... not really."

Them: "You think it's normal if it happens?"

Me: "Uh ... I'm not a urologist."

QUESTION TWO

> Them: "Hey, we're about the same age, right?"
>
> Me (dreading this): "Yeah."
>
> Them: "You ever notice that you don't have as many orgasms when you have sex as you used to?"
>
> Me: "Well, it's not like when I was eighteen."
>
> Them: "So you think it's normal?"
>
> Me: "Uh … I'm not a urologist."

QUESTION THREE

> Them: "Hey, we're about the same age, right?"
>
> Me (dreading this): "Yeah."
>
> Them: "You ever notice your pee stream is not as strong as it used to be?"
>
> Me: *"Go see a damn urologist!"*

But it's not just physical stuff. Clients want to tell me every intimate detail of their personal lives.

I've had female clients tell me that they're planning to divorce their husbands and take off with the kids. Then I see their husbands, who I'm also training, and they literally have no idea that their world is about to be turned upside down.

One husband kept telling me about all the hookers he brought into his office because his wife wouldn't sleep with him. Meanwhile, when I'm working out with his wife, she says her husband has no sexual interest in her, but that she's interested in me. She tried to seduce me every time I went there, even going so far as to show up dressed in a miniskirt, stripper heels and bustier. Not exactly appropriate gear for the treadmill. She turned up the music and proceeded to start what could only be described as a lap dance. I have a steadfast rule not to get involved with clients and told her so. She ended up apologizing and we never brought it up again.

But, most of the time, along with the workouts, I'm a friendly ear and a shoulder to cry on. Clients often can't wait to tell me everything that's going on in their lives, so much so that I have trouble remembering it all.

"They said yes!" a client might chirp as I walk through the door.

"Great!" I reply, trying to remember exactly who was supposed to say yes to what.

To some clients, I'm the go-to guy about everything.

In 1994, I was in Aspen when the big Northridge earthquake hit L.A. As soon as it happened, I got calls from three different clients all asking me the same question. What should I do? I had to explain to them that I'm from Louisiana and don't have much in the way of earthquake training.

And not only do I become the go-to guy, I often become part of the family.

The kids of many of my clients start calling me "Uncle Vinnie" and want me to go watch them during a baseball game or see them in a play. And sometimes I go.

I usually have the keys to my clients' houses and the codes to their alarms. I've gotten calls at two in the morning from clients who got locked out of their homes and need me to drive over and let them in. I always do.

One guy told a friend of his that hiring me was the best deal he ever made because his wife dropped her shrink soon after she started working out with me.

I can understand why.

I show up on time. I'm reliable. I pay attention.

I know when a client is scared, vulnerable or upset and needs some handholding. This is when I go into my "love me, daddy" mode.

I know when a client is in a type-A mood and wants to jump into the workout in a clinical "just the facts, ma'am" kind of way. I can do that.

I know when clients need motivation and want me to supply it, which means I go into my "you're the man!" routine.

I love my job. In fact, I love it for the very reasons most people find it bizarre. I love that I don't have an office to go to, or a 9 to 5 schedule. I love that I might have an extra hour to go out for a jog. I love that I don't have to shave every day. Some days I'm as clean cut as a marine, other days I'm as scraggly as a bum. In fact, the longer I go without shaving, the cooler my clients think I am. I love that exercise is built into my job. On any given day, I'm hiking up a mountain with this client, running four miles through town with that one and biking sixty miles over a canyon with another one.

Most trainers will limit a client to an hour per session. I'm from Louisiana and we have a term there called "lagniappe." It means "a little something extra." If a bartender fills your glass to the top, that's lagniappe. When I charge someone for an appointment, I give them lagniappe. I call it a single session even if we go much longer because I want them to get their money's worth. Hell, I've taken clients out for six-hour bike rides.

Like I said, I don't do this job for the money.

From my point of view, I provide a service that's unmatched by anyone. A real pro trainer has to be a combination of running coach, weight-lifting coach, nutritionist, stretching instructor, amateur orthopedist, motivational speaker and life counselor.

I'm proud of what I do.

I have a top fitness podcast you can find on iTunes (just search for Vinnie Tortorich) and on my website (www.vinnietortorich.com). I start each episode by saying, "Your good intentions have been stolen and I'm here to help you get them back," because it pisses me off when people try to get fit, only to quit in frustration after a shitty diet or worthless supplement or useless piece of gear has let them down.

Again.

I usually train the rich and famous but now I want you to think of me as *your* trainer. I've spent decades helping people get fit and now I'm going to help you. And, when we're done, you're going to know how to get in better shape than you've ever been in your life.

I'll teach you the right way to exercise and diet (hint: don't diet.) Maybe you've never exercised a day in your life. Maybe you've tried a hundred diets and failed a hundred times. Maybe your house looks like a garage sale filled with unused *Gut Busters* and *Sweatin' to the Oldies* tapes.

Don't worry.

I got this.

During the course of our adventure together, I'm going to give you tons of helpful hints. I'll tell you the single best piece of fitness equipment ever invented—and it's affordable to everyone. I'll tell you which is more important to losing weight, diet or exercise (and, no, the answer isn't "it's both!") I'll show you the exercises that give you the most bang for your buck.

Remember, I'm your personal trainer now.

Over the years, I've had great success, but I don't measure it in dollar bills. Most people use money as a means of keeping score. I think that's crap. By that measure, a guy who wins the lottery is the most successful guy in the world instead of a loser who just bought a bunch of tickets.

The only thing money's good for is to buy stuff, and who needs all that stuff? Hell, at fifty years old, I don't own a home, a couch or a television and the last time I wore underwear was in high school. My mom calls me eccentric. My friends think I'm "colorful." I think I'm perfectly normal. Whenever I move, I do it in one carload.

So how do I measure success? I measure it by the success of my clients. If they've reached their goals, then I feel successful. If they surpass those goals, I feel like I've hit the lottery. Tickets purchased? Zero.

Let's get started.

Part One

EAT TO LOSE

Chapter Two
OBESITY

IT'S A PROBLEM. You don't need me to tell you that people in this country are fat and getting fatter. Hell, they just redid the "It's A Small World" ride at Disneyland. Know why? They had to make the waterways that hold the boats deeper because the weight of today's passengers made the things bottom out and get stuck. They should rename it "It's A Fat World."

Fat is everywhere!

Turn on the TV. It's all about fat. If it's a morning show, there's no shortage of people telling Matt Lauer how to get rid of it. By mid-day, Jerry and Maury have the fat people fighting each other like they're in a circus side-show. By mid-afternoon, you have Ricki Lake either gaining a hundred pounds or losing a hundred. By the time you get to the six o'clock news, they're calling it an epidemic. In primetime, they've created games to lose it.

And what do we put in between all that fat?

Commercials.

Commercials for diet food. Commercials for supplements. Commercials for fitness products. Commercials for prescription drugs that promise to do everything from lower our cholesterol to get rid of our high blood pressure to cure our sleep apnea—all things that would usually go away naturally if we weren't fat. And, when all that stuff fails, then come the commercials for gastric by-pass surgery. These guys want to perform surgery on us because they don't think we can be trusted with a digestive tract!

Does any of this stuff work? No! And they know it doesn't.

Study after study shows that none of that stuff is effective long term, not even cutting out your stomach. Hell, if it did work, we'd all be getting thinner, but just the opposite is happening. And do you think the businesses that profit from this care?

Of course they do.

As long as you stay fat.

They don't want you thin, because if you're thin they can't make any more money off you. But it can't be their fault that their products don't work, because then they'd look like the frauds they are, so they have to blame it on something else—so they picked a clown. That's right, these geniuses want us to blame McDonald's and other fast food companies for their shortcomings!

Let's get real.

McDonald's and those other fast food chains are not guilty of making us fat. The only thing they're guilty of is making meat taste bad which is why they use white bread and sugary ketchup to sexy it up. Don't believe me? Order a fast food burger and just eat the meat. You have a better chance of finishing *War And Peace*. Whatever happened to personal responsibility? You know who thinks McDonald's is health food?

No one.

Let's take cigarettes. There was a time when cigarettes didn't have any warnings on the package. In fact, there were even com-mercials that showed doctors smoking while talking about how soothing they are to your throat. But even with all that, as a young kid I knew cigarettes had to be bad for you. How? One night I was sitting by a campfire and the wind started blowing the smoke into my face. I was miserable. My eyes began to water, I started choking. So you know what I did? I got up and moved to the other side of the campfire.

Problem solved.

To smoke is the equivalent of sitting on the smoky side of a campfire. Who in their right mind would do that? We know it's bad for us, yet we do it anyway.

Fast food is the same way.

We know we shouldn't eat it, but we do. And then we pretend to be surprised when some moron makes a movie "exposing" how bad it is for us. Remember that movie? It was called *Super-Size Me* and it starred that idiot with the facial hair that makes him look like a seventies porn star.

We shouldn't blame McDonald's when we get fat. But now that many of us are, who should we turn to in order to help us lose the weight?

I'll tell you who we shouldn't turn to—Jenny Craig. You know what business Jenny is in? You think it's the weight loss business? You think it's the diet business?

Think again.

Our good friend Jenny is in the food service industry.

Why do you think it costs almost nothing to join? Jenny and her buddies over at Weight Watchers and Nutrisystem want to keep it cheap, or even free, on the sign-up to get you in the door. They don't make money off their program, they make it by selling you their food.

You're probably asking "don't people lose weight on those diets?"

Sure. Of course they do. And that's good and fine as long as you plan on counting "points" or eating their pre-packaged crap for the rest of your life, which means no tiramasu for you ... ever.

There's a better way.

You can lose weight faster than on these diet programs and be completely sated without the tyranny of spending your entire life eating freeze-dried, engineered garbage.

But before we get into that, how did we become an obese nation?

Years ago, I was at a Springsteen concert in the New Orleans Superdome when the Boss said something in that familiar growl of his that stuck with me.

"I've been doing this for twenty five years," he said, "and I stand up here and look out into the audience and see the same faces year after year. And I realize that my audience is getting older but I still stay the same!"

Well, that line came back to me when I went to my twentieth high school reunion. I was trying to find a parking spot when I noticed some older folks walking into the restaurant where it was taking place. I mentioned to my friend, Todd, that it was nice they invited some of the parents to the reunion. Todd shook his head and said, "Man those aren't the parents … those are our classmates!"

I was shocked. They looked closer to people in their late fifties than late thirties. I sat outside in the car for the next fifteen minutes, watching people walk in, and I became obsessed with trying to figure out why they looked so much older than they really were.

Finally, it dawned on me.

They were fat. It wasn't just gut and love handles. Their faces were jowly. Many had double chins. And the way the extra weight made them move, ponderous and slow, as if they were struggling uphill, also added to the illusion of age. And it wasn't just a few of them … it was most of them.

How did this happen?

How did we get here?

Almost everyone in my family, aside from me, is fat and, in some cases, morbidly obese. But it wasn't always that way. My grandparents on both sides were thin, not to mention their brothers and sisters. They were all lean and healthy, most of them living into their nineties and carrying no extra weight to their deathbeds. There was no heart disease to speak of. No diabetes.

Did they exercise? Not in a gym, not the way we do now. But they weren't lazy people. They did all their own yard work. They tended their own vegetable gardens, some as big as five acres. They were active.

What about their diets?

Here's a typical breakfast. Because we were in Southern Louisiana, grits were generally available but they were the exception, not the rule. My grandparent's breakfast was always the same. Bacon and eggs. The eggs were fried in butter, not margarine. The bacon came from a pig, where it's supposed to come from. Not from a ground-up turkey with "bacon-like" flavoring added. Along with the breakfast, they drank coffee with cream in it.

No skinny lattes there.

For lunch, it was a full-cooked meal. A stewed chicken. Roast beef. Maybe flank steak. As a side dish, they had some veggies sautéed in butter. And if the veggies were raw, they were made into an antipasto, with deli meats and tons of good olive oil mixed in. If there was any gravy or oil left on a plate, they might use a half piece of bread to soak it up.

Dinner was the same. Might have been leftovers from lunch or, more likely, fish because fish was reserved for the evenings and was plentiful in Louisiana. As a side dish, maybe a little bit of rice or a couple spoonfuls of pasta. To drink? Water, usually. Or, on my mom's side, maybe some wine.

For dessert? They didn't have dessert although, occasionally, they might have a scoop of ice cream as a special treat. Nowadays, kids get dessert as a reward for eating everything on their plate. Let me break that down for you. The reward for over-eating is to get to over-eat even more.

And what about snacking? The closest my grandparents ever came to snacking was when my grandfather might lop off a piece of cheese from the fridge and nibble at it.

In other words, back then, their diets consisted of fried eggs, bacon, beef and other meats, cream, butter, whole milk, vegetables and fruit. Sound crazy? How could you possibly lose weight on a diet like that?

The answer? They never lost weight on a diet like that.

Because they never gained weight to begin with.

Did they learn this way of eating from a book? Or television? No, they learned it from their parents. And guess where their parents came from?

Italy.

Amazingly, I actually knew my great grandparents, because most of them lived close to their hundredth birthday, never having had high blood pressure, cholesterol problems or diabetes.

How did they stay so healthy? To find the answer, let's talk about Europe for a minute.

People are always obsessed with Italy and France. Why are those people so thin? It seems impossible. We think of Frenchmen as eating baguettes all the time, mostly because whenever we see them in movies, they're carrying a grocery bag with a baguette sticking out of it. But you know what they don't eat a lot of in France?

Bread.

Here's what they do eat. Meats cooked in olive oil and butter. Cheese everywhere. My God, the French love their cheese! They even serve it for dessert. And they put cream on everything. Hell, they came up with *crème fraiche*. But you know what the French didn't come up with? French fries and French vanilla ice cream.

You know who did?

We did.

Let's talk about the Italians. We all know what they eat. Pasta, right! Think again. They eat exactly like my grandparents did.

Pasta is usually just a side-dish, not the main course. They also eat a lot of antipasto (meats and cheeses) and they love their olives, which seem to taste better over there for some reason. You know what else tastes better in Italy?

Ice cream!

Those Italians love their ice cream. And you know why it tastes better over there? Because they don't believe in fat-free ice cream. As a matter of fact, they like to double the cream content, which leaves a lot less room for sugar. They call it gelato, their own invention. But you know what the Italians didn't invent?

Pizza!

You know who did?

We did.

In the past half-century, Americans have been getting fatter while the Europeans stayed thin. Until recently. Studies have shown that the Europeans are catching up to us on the scales.

The reason is not really a mystery.

More and more, Europeans are eating Americanized diets. Remember those French fries that the French didn't invent and the pizza that the Italians didn't invent? The Europeans are now eating them, too, along with all the other crap we consume, like pre-packaged meals, Big Gulps, bags of chips, you name it.

And it's not just the adults.

When I first moved to L.A., I was greeted with a whole new group of clientele. Kids. Desperate parents with obese eleven and twelve year olds wanted me to take the weight off them. Fifty pounds. A hundred pounds. It was shocking. And that trend has only grown. Today, over half of my clients are children. How did they get so fat?

Trying to be healthy!

Their parents have been told over and over that kids need to eat their vitamins, so what do they find on store shelves? Vitamins—inside gummy bears! Or in the shape of a Flintstone—made out of sugar!

Look on breakfast cereal boxes. Does this sound familiar? "Provides 8 essential vitamins and iron." That sounds healthy, right? Know what cereal that was on?

Honey Smacks! Healthy old Honey Smacks!

That's like adding vitamins to plutonium so you can claim atomic bombs are good for you. And since we're on the subject of Honey Smacks, let's talk about this wonderful product. Did you know that Consumer Reports said it was tied (with Golden Crisps) for highest sugar content in a breakfast cereal? Want to know what percentage of Honey Smacks is sugar?

Over fifty percent.

Advocacy groups were calling Kellog's out on this fact and they got an interesting reply. According to CNN, Linda Sutherland, Kellog's vice president of nutrition, explained that Honey Smacks is not marketed to children.

Let's think about that for a second.

You know what's on the cover of a box of Honey Smacks? Dig'em Frog. A big green smiling cartoon frog.

To be fair, other notable mascots used to sell Honey Smacks to "adults" include Cliffy the Clown, Smaxey the Seal, Wally the Bear and Quick Draw McGraw. Now, I don't know about you, but those cartoon characters don't exactly seem designed to hook grown-ups. I have yet to be at a business breakfast and hear an executive say, "Let's see, why don't you have eggs benedict while I go with a bowl of Honey Smacks."

And if you're sitting there reading this and thinking, "Honey Smacks sounds familiar, but didn't it used to be called *Sugar* Smacks?" give yourself a gold star. Kellog's changed the name in the eighties. I'm guessing it's because "Honey" sounded healthier. That's the same reason Kentucky Fried Chicken became KFC after people became aware of how terrible fried foods are for you.

But enough about breakfast cereal. What's the other thing parents are told to give their kids because it's good for them?

Fruit!

Remember when fruit used to mean apples and oranges and bananas? Now we have fruit roll-ups, where they literally take out everything that's great about the fruit and leave you with a slab of sugar.

This isn't new, by the way.

Remember Tang? That's what was around when I was a kid. It was basically a glass full of colored sugar. And why do you think our parents thought this was good for us? Because it had vitamins in it. And you want to know why *we* drank it? Because the astronauts drank it. It was created by a guy named William Mitchell. Would you like to know what other healthy products this genius invented?

Pop Rocks, Cool Whip and instant-set Jell-O.

Look, if we don't know better, how can we expect our kids to? Truth is, I really like working with kids because they're not so set in their ways and they're willing to listen when I tell them how to eat to stay thin and fit. They always want to know what diet they should go on. I love to hear that, because it gives me the opportunity to stop them from a lifetime of yo-yo-ing through one bad diet after another.

So I give them the secret to going on a diet. Here it is.

Don't.

Chapter Three
THE NON-DIET

WHENEVER I ASK people how they're eating, they usually tell me one of two things:

"Ooooh, I've been good!"
OR
"Ooooh, I've been bad."

"Good" meaning that they're depriving themselves of food. "Bad" meaning that they're actually eating.

This flies in the face of what every other species in the animal kingdom does on a daily basis, where a good day is when they actually get something to eat and a bad one is when they go hungry. Can you imagine a lion telling his cubs, "Hey kids, great news! I let that zebra go. I'm sorry you're all gonna starve but, hey, we're being good!"

Insane, right?

But that's what we do. And we've even come up with a word for it: "diet." You know how the dictionary defines diet? As the kinds of food that a person, animal, or community habitually eats.

Unfortunately, it doesn't mean that anymore, at least not to most people. We've now bastardized the term to mean deprivation, starvation and suffering.

We think of a diet as something short-term, something with an ending, something with an expiration date. And, usually, we have a clear goal. Say you want to lose twenty pounds, so you go on a diet. You're doing pretty good, limiting your food, denying yourself ... but then you get tested. You're getting your car tuned up at the dealership when they bring out the free doughnuts. But these are not just your basic powdered sugar jobs. It's a cornucopia of temptation.

Doughnut holes dipped in vanilla icing and rolled in sprinkles. The éclair covered in chocolate with just the right amount of Bavarian cream bursting from the side. And let's not forget the cruller. Oh, the cruller. A doughnut strategically designed to hold more sugar than any other. The cruller is a masterpiece, the perfect storm of doughnut. In the interest of full disclosure, I've fallen prey to the cruller several times. It's no accident that "cruller" sounds suspiciously like "crueler."

But it doesn't matter what shape or form the doughnuts come in, they're all the same thing—instant fat pills. Even though you know this, you still want one ... but, heroically, you resist.

You walk out of that dealership with a fresh oil change and tire rotation, along with a sense of empowerment. You've fought the cruller ... and won! And you know what you thought you were being?

Good.

And it's easy to be good because you know you only have to do it for a short time. Why? Because eventually you're going to reach your goal weight and the heavens will part, and the angels will sing, and your diet will finally be over. And once that happens, you'll be so happy with your new body that you'll tell yourself, "I will never go back to my old way of eating."

But you have no choice.

You were able to gut through the diet for a limited time because you had a specific goal in mind. You could be good for a while.

But now it's dinner time.

And the food looks great. It's the first non pre-packaged meal you've seen in months. Lasagna. And breaded veal. And look at those buttered rolls on the table! You know they're hot without even touching them because you can smell the heat.

And that's when it dawns on you—this isn't on your diet. And if you can't go back to your old way of eating, you can't eat it. And that's when you start talking to yourself.

"Wait a minute … is this what I signed up for?"

"You mean I have to count calories … forever?"

"I have to eat pre-packaged rice bars … for all eternity?"

"I'm supposed to drink special herb tea … until I die?"

Screw this, you think!

So you start making deals with yourself. You know what I'm talking about. You've been there.

I'll just have it tonight.

Only this once, to celebrate being back at my high school weight.

What's life worth if I can't have a little fun sometimes?

I'll just eat the dinner … but not the dessert.

So you do that. You eat the dinner knowing you're planning to skip the dessert and just have a cup of coffee. But then the dessert comes, the one everyone else is going to eat.

And it's bread pudding.

Shit. You promised you were going to be good with the dessert, but you're only human! And they put a buttery, whisky sauce on it. A sugary, buttery, whisky sauce. You beat the cruller in the car dealership but this is cruel and unusual punishment! Do they really expect you to beat the cruller forever?

What is this restaurant, the Spanish inquisition?

Screw this, you think. You're in charge of your own life and you're eating the bread pudding, damnit!

And, right then and there, even though you won't admit it to yourself, you know deep down inside that you're sunk.

A few months later, you find yourself not just twenty pounds heavier, but thirty. But you think you know why. You realize that you'd just been on the wrong diet. So which diet should you try now?

The cabbage soup diet?

Maybe the Cambridge?

Or maybe you should just do one of the many cleanse diets and starve yourself for a few days.

It's so hard. Which to choose? But wait—here's one you haven't heard of before. Eating for your blood type. That's it. That's why the last diet failed. You weren't eating for your blood type!

Now that you know the proper diet, you're certain you can quickly drop this thirty pounds and never go back to your old way of eating again.

Problem solved, right?

Of course not. You're now on what I call the "diet treadmill." You get on it, run for miles and, when you get off, you discover you haven't moved an inch. It's frustrating. You feel like a failure. And all the big diet companies perpetuate that by telling you that you failed because you stupidly picked the wrong diet. In other words, not their diet. But when their diet fails you, they make you feel like it's your fault by saying you just didn't have the willpower to follow it properly.

I got news for you.

Nobody has the willpower to starve.

This is why I don't want you to diet, because they don't work long term. Not only that, many of them are flat out ludicrous. Years ago, I was dating the anchorwoman of the six o'clock news in New Orleans and she did a story on the worst diets ever. Here are a few of them.

The "Prayer Diet" where, instead of eating, you prayed.

The "Sludge Diet" where you ate fast food, pizza and ice cream to create a "sludge" in your body that supposedly drew away the fat.

The "Chocolate Diet" which was similar to the "Sludge Diet" except you did it with chocolate.

She finished her report by saying that these diets wouldn't work under any circumstances and, in some cases, could be harmful to your health. You know what happened? In those pre-Google days, the station was inundated with calls from desperate people frantic to know more about how they could get on those diets. The very ones she just said were harmful!

Things are even worse today.

Remember when they took the diet drug Fen-Phen off the market because it was giving people strokes and causing them to drop dead? People went apeshit. But they weren't upset that it was killing people, they were upset that it was taken away. Sure, there was a chance you might die but so what? You lost weight, didn't you?

People are willing to die to be thin. They want the secret. They want it now.

I'm a guy in the trenches. I deal with celebrities every day who have to stay fit to get jobs and pay their mortgage. They also can't show up on set tired and lethargic. For twenty years, I've been helping them and now I'm going to help you by sharing the same weight-loss secret. Here it is.

STAY AWAY FROM SUGAR AND GRAINS

Let me tell you what you're feeling right now: a big let-down.

You didn't know what I was going to say, but you were hoping it was some kind of trick you'd never heard before. But even though you may not realize it yet, what I just told you is magical. If you just do it, if you just—

STAY AWAY FROM SUGAR
and
STAY AWAY FROM GRAINS

—then you are going to be thin. It's that simple. Notice what I didn't say.

I didn't say you need to count calories.

I didn't say you need to eat low fat.

I didn't say you had to watch your portions.

I didn't say you need to exercise an hour a day.

The reason I didn't say you need to do those things is because *you are not on a diet.*

I'm always able to tell when a new client will fail at losing weight long term when they ask me "how long will it take me to lose this weight?" I have a standard Vinnie-ism I give them in reply.

"Why? Are you going to stop when you get there?"

Whenever I hear that question, I know the client has a finish line in mind.

You don't.

Life's not like one of those TV weight-loss shows like *Biggest Loser* or *Heavy*. We can't leave home for months at a time and be whisked off to a fatless fairyland where elves deliver us the perfect calorie-controlled meals, and trainers attend to us 24/7 for free. The truth is, if you look at the meals they serve on those shows the contestants are basically on starvation diets, which is not sustainable in the real world.

The camera loves it when you get a five hundred pound guy to drop a couple hundred pounds fast. Unfortunately, they're setting them up for failure because they've got to leave paradise at some point and once the lights are off and the cameras are gone, these people have to find a way to live and eat like that for the rest of their lives.

Not you.

You are about to make a lifestyle change that is going to allow you to shed weight quickly and naturally, without pain and suffering, in a way that you will be able to easily maintain. I know you won't just take my word for it, because it sounds too simple to be true, so I'm going to explain it a little more.

Don't worry.

I'm not a scientist, so I promise not to get too sciency on you. There are plenty of books out there that do that very well, and I'll point you in their direction if you're interested. What I am going to do is explain why this works in a way that even I can understand.

Then I'm going to show you how to do it.

But before we get into that, we need to confront something head on. The myth of calories in, calories out.

Chapter Four
WHY CALORIES IN,
CALORIES OUT IS BULLSHIT

BACK IN THE eighties, you couldn't find a school, gym or church hall that didn't have an aerobics class. Jane Fonda went from movie star to fitness expert overnight, and polyester got a new name. Spandex. They had to do something with it, the seventies were over and no one was buying leisure suits any more. I had to see for myself what this craze was all about, so I checked out an aerobics class.

The instructor barked instructions over the sound of Abba's *Dancing Queen*, which blared from the boombox. "Squeeze your buns! Feel the burn!" And, my favorite: "Breathe!" Just in case we'd forgotten to. "We're burning calories!" she'd say. "Only twenty more calories and we can get rid of that cheesecake! Only ten more minutes of calorie burning and you can have a scoop of ice cream! There's thirty-four hundred calories in a pound of fat!"

She drove me crazy, in spite of how hot she was. She was a dancing calorie-counting abacus, even though she was making it all up as she went along. When the class was over, I decided to have some fun with her, along with trying to get a date.

"That was a lot of great information you gave us," I said. "But I do have a question. What's a calorie?"

You could almost see the question mark above her head as she puzzled through that.

"What do you mean?" she asked.

"Well, you had a lot to say about calories so I was just wondering … what's a calorie?"

"Oh. A calorie is a thing you eat."

"Really?" I said. "I thought that was called food."

She hemmed and hawed and I finally decided to let her off the hook. "A calorie," I told her, "is a unit of heat. It's the amount of heat required to raise the temperature of one gram of water by one degree Celsius."

She answered by offering me a piece of fitness gum, the kind that promised to get you into shape just by chewing it. I took the gum and realized I'd probably lost her at the word "heat." The point is, we all talk about calories, but not many of us know exactly what they are. Actually, I could have just started by saying that, but then I wouldn't have gotten to tell you that I hooked up with the aerobics instructor.

Anyway. Even though not everyone is completely sure what a calorie is, it's commonly accepted that too many of them makes us fat unless we get rid of them. This is usually known as the calorie in, calorie out concept. The idea, drummed into us year after year, is that to lose weight you have to burn more calories than you consume.

The simplicity of this is part of its appeal. Does it work? Well, it can. If, over time, you take in fewer calories than you expend, you will lose weight as long as your calories come mainly in the form of fat and protein. But if most of your calories come from carbohydrates, you will lose less weight. The idea that a "calorie is a calorie" is false, because your body reacts differently to different kinds of calories, but we'll get into that later.

The other problem with the calorie in, calorie out concept is that it's based on trickery. We're forcing ourselves to go against what our bodies naturally want us to do, which is eat, not starve. If you want to understand why calorie in, calorie out is flawed as a weight-loss strategy, look no further than your nearest triathlon.

Let's play a game.

Picture in your mind the type of person that completes a triathlon. I'm guessing you're visualizing a lean, muscular athlete. And, if you look at the top pros featured in the magazines, you'd think that everyone who completes a triathlon looks exactly like that.

But let's ignore them for a second. Let's look at everyone else, the people who complete the triathlon but are not in the top third. Would you agree that anyone who can complete a triathlon is in prime physical shape? Remember, you have to train hard enough to be able to swim 2.2 miles in open water, immediately followed by 112 miles on a bicycle, immediately followed by running a full 26.2 mile marathon.

Any one of these feats by themselves is heroic. Put them together and it's almost inconceivable to the average person. So, by anyone's definition, these contestants would have to be among the most fit human beings on the planet. And aerobically they might be.

But they don't always look it.

How do I know? Because I always stay to the end of these competitions. That's where the real human drama is. Sure, we all admire the pros who do it in record time, but what about the regular folks, the people who have trained as many hours as the pros and are in it to prove to themselves that they can do something that seems impossible? At the end of the competition, between the fifteenth and seventeenth hour, you see the true triumph of the human spirit. People who are literally willing their bodies across the finish line just to prove they can.

I love these people. Watching them is like being in a quadruple feature of *Rudy*, *Rocky*, *Something For Joey* and *Brian's Song*. So I know what I'm talking about when I say that these folks, the back-of-the-packers, the ones with something to prove, these folks are often carrying extra weight on them. And not just a little.

How is that possible?

Can you imagine the amount of calories they expend training for this? Hundreds of thousands. By the pure calorie in, calorie out theory, they should all be rail thin, but they're not. So why the disparity?

Because what pros do and what they say they do are two different things.

Understand this—pros, in order to survive financially, have to have sponsorships. Gatorade, Power Bar, Gu. There's no shortage of companies willing to pay them money to publicly endorse and use their products. And the pros do use their products ... when the cameras are on them or the fans are around. But Gatorade and all the other sport drink companies make fundamentally the same thing: sugar water. The only thing that differentiates it from soda is carbonation.

The pros know this.

And they also know that, in order to secure these sponsorships, they need to win races and stay lean. But if they spend their days drinking sugar water, it's going to be tough to keep the weight off. So they take a few sips for the benefit of the public but, in private, they know enough to quench their thirst with water, hydration we still haven't improved on. By the way, that reminds me of a Vinnie-ism.

> *You want to know where you can find the fountain of youth?*
> *Look in a fountain.*

The same thing holds true for Power Bars and all the other sport-type bars. They're full of sugar, not to mention, in many cases, partially hydrogenated oils, which make them about as nutritious as a candy bar. Again, in public, you'll see the pros nibble but, in private, they'll try to get their carbohydrates from fruits and vegetables.

Same holds true for all the goops and sports gels that promise to give you "sustained energy." Again, they're all sugar. The pros eat them for the cameras and during long endurance events, but during training, they eat proper diets. High protein, high fat along with some carbs.

In fact, if you ate the way the pros pretend to eat to satisfy their sponsors, you could eat healthier at an eight-year-old's birthday party. If you think I'm kidding, recently the Jelly Belly company started marketing "sports beans" which are just jelly beans with a few vitamins thrown in. The pros won't touch them. Why?

Because pros know nothing will shut you down quicker than sugar.

But let's get back to our amateur triathletes. They don't necessarily know all this. They drink the Gatorade, they eat the power bars and they buy into the concept of "carb-loading" where you eat nothing but pasta, bread and rice for days on end to give you "energy." They've trained like champions and have brought themselves physically and mentally to a place where they can complete a triathlon, but their diet has left them, in some cases, heavier than when they started, in spite of the fact that they've expended hundreds of thousands of calories during their training. Usually, they themselves are baffled by their weight gain.

I can't begin to tell you how many calls I've gotten from amateurs in the middle of training for a triathlon, desperate to know how they can possibly be gaining weight. And when I tell them why, you know how they usually react?

They don't believe me, because they've spent years being conditioned by magazine ads and commercials to think that they're doing it the right way. The truth is, our bodies react differently to different kinds of calories, which is why the simple calorie in, calorie out concept is fundamentally flawed. So let's talk about how your body reacts to calories from sugars and grains, which will help you understand why they're killing you.

Chapter Five
THE FOOD PYRAMID SCHEME

FIRST OF ALL, when I say grains, what am I talking about? Wheat, corn and rice. And not just in their pure form, but in any product where they're used. Bread, pasta and crackers are just a few of the grain-based foods that are generally thought of as being good for you. They're also the basis of a million other products that we instinctively know aren't good for us, like pop-tarts, corn chips and kid's breakfast cereals.

And those are just the products that are obvious about it. There are a ton of others that are a lot sneakier.

Grains are used as fillers in most processed foods, like ready-to-eat microwaveable meals and frozen entrees. Even more insidious is when they're converted into sugar. Ever wonder what high fructose corn syrup or maltodextrine is? It's corn that's been chemically altered to turn it into a sweetener. You'll find it in candy bars and pasta sauce and most other processed foods.

And when they can't get us to chew it any more, they get us to drink it.

The sugar in soda? In most cases, it's high fructose corn syrup. Remember those sports drinks we were talking about?

Check the labels. I bet you find high fructose corn syrup in a majority of them.

But what's really so bad about sugar and grain? Why is a calorie from them different from any other calorie?

It's different because your body processes it differently. Since the dawn of man, we were designed to handle protein, fat and natural carbohydrates because that's what was naturally around us. That's what the cavemen ate to survive. What they didn't eat was the crap we have now—processed carbs and sugar. In fact, you want to know why we're born with a sweet tooth?

To save our lives.

Poisonous plants usually have a bitter taste in contrast to the sweet-ish taste of the ones that aren't deadly. Our natural sweet tooth was designed to be a line of defense to steer us away from the plants that could kill us. But nowadays, if you were to turn a caveman loose in a grocery store, he'd think he was in heaven and eat himself into a diabetic coma without ever realizing he was actually swallowing poison.

After a couple hundred thousand years of our bodies processing the foods they were designed to process, the last two decades have seen us flood our bodies with carbs and sugar. Will we eventually evolve to be able to deal with that stuff? Maybe, in another hundred thousand years or so. But, for right now, we have a problem. We're getting fat.

You want to know what I blame for this?

The food pyramid!

You've seen this ridiculous thing. Since the early nineties, the USDA has been telling us that the foundation for any nutritious diet is grain, which they show as the base of the pyramid. The whole thing is nothing but a pyramid scheme. They've been asking us to buy into this bullshit high-carb lifestyle for decades but it's now finally collapsing under the weight of all the Americans who've gotten fat as a result!

But that can't be true, you say. Because if it is, that means the government is wrong.

Guess what? They know they are. That's why they recently re-did the pyramid and removed some of the grain that they want you to eat. But not enough. Not even close. And there's a reason for that. We're supposed to have checks and balances in this country, right? Would you like to know who checks on the USDA?

The USDA.

That's right, they answer only to themselves. There's no balance there, but there sure are plenty of checks—being written to farmers. Since the Great Depression, the US has been paying farmers to grow grain to keep the economy going, because back then it was agriculturally based. But all these years later, we're still doing it, which means we're producing huge amounts of grain. We don't want to let it go to waste, so we've found ways to use it in every corner of our lives. Our food, our beverages, even our gas tanks.

The truth is, it was all pretty harmless when it was just a little extra corn and bread. Our bodies could handle it. But, over time, it's ended up in everything. Like the Kardashians. And now that we're flooded with that garbage in such unprecedented quantities, our bodies don't know what to do with it and so we convert it to fat and store it.

That's the simple answer. The more complicated one involves how sugar and grain is immediately converted to glucose once it hits your bloodstream, which triggers the release of insulin, which begins the process of storing the glucose as fat in your cells.

If that sentence bored you when you read it, don't feel alone. It bored me to write it. But if you're interested in learning more, there are plenty of great books out there by scientists and doctors that go into this in detail. *Why We Get Fat And What To Do About It* by Gary Taubes is good. So is *The Art And Science Of Low Carbohydrate Living* by Dr. Stephen Phinney, along with *Fat Chance: Beating the Odds Against Sugar, Processed Food, Obesity, and Disease* by Dr. Robert H. Lustig.

What's important to understand is that sugars and grains enter your body and are stored as fat. You don't want that.

But they give me energy, you might say.

For a few minutes, yeah, until you crash. You can get all the short-term energy you need from the unprocessed sugar in the fiber of natural fruits and vegetables. The fiber slows down its absorption into your bloodstream, preventing that nasty glucose-insulin spike, giving you all the short-term energy benefits but not the fat-storing downside.

And if that wasn't enough reason to hate sugar and grains, they screw you in another way. Hunger. The second they enter your body, your blood sugar spikes, which makes you feel great. You know the feeling. You've been there. It's like a drug. But that spike is followed by a crash and it leaves you jonesing for more.

In other words, you get hungry.

So you eat more carbs. Chips, another slice of pizza, one more scoop of ice cream. This triggers another spike, followed by another crash. It's a vicious cycle, not unlike a cigarette or heroin addiction. And each time this happens, you're taking your body on an insulin roller coaster and storing more and more fat.

Speaking of fat, what happens when we eat fat? Does it make us more fat? Seems like it would if we believe the theory that "you are what you eat." But we know that's not true. Eating a chicken doesn't make you grow feathers. That reminds me of another Vinnie-ism.

The biggest problem with fat is that it's called fat.

Just like being out in the cold doesn't give you a cold, eating fat doesn't make you fat. We've taken the word fat and demonized it to the point that it sounds as bad as the other F-word. Come on, give fat a break! It's not fat's fault it's called fat! So what is it then?

Energy.

At least that's how our body recognizes it. In fact, let's pretend for a second that we call fat something different. Let's change the word "fat" to "energy." Then, when we're enjoying an avocado or a nice steak or a cheese platter, we wouldn't think of these foods as being fattening, we'd think of them as being "energizing."

Fat is actually our body's preferred long-term energy source. Not only that, because it doesn't trigger the insulin whiplash that sugars and grains do, you don't have spikes and crashes, which means you don't stay hungry all the time. In fact, it's not unusual for people eating a high fat lifestyle to completely lose their sugar cravings and miss a meal.

In fact, you want to demonize something. How about this? Teflon! Before Teflon was invented, we cooked foods in regular pans with butter, oil and lard. You heard me, lard! And you know what that did? Besides keeping the food from sticking to your pan, it added flavor and something even more crucial—more fat, AKA more energy.

Plus, it made you feel sated.

Let's say you had some egg whites for breakfast, cooked in a non-stick Teflon coated pan that required absolutely no fat. You remember what it tasted like? Crap. Did it fill you up? No. You were still hungry afterwards, which made you want to eat more food. By 9 a.m. you were thinking about the vending machine at work and by 10 you were digesting a Snickers to tide you over till lunch.

Thanks, Teflon.

So let's talk protein. How does protein fit into this whole scheme if fat is what we use for long-term energy? Protein is what we use to rebuild our bodies after normal daily wear and tear breaks us down. Every cell in the human body is built on protein. Your hair, your organs, your muscles, even your baby blues. We need it to live, and the best way to get it is naturally in the form of meat, poultry, fish, eggs and dairy products.

So if fat is used for long-term energy and carbohydrates from fruits and vegetables are used for short-term energy and protein is used to rebuild our cells, what is sugar and grain used for?

Getting us fat.

If you don't eat them, the only thing you have to lose is weight. If you simply stay away from sugar and grains, the weight will come flying off. Hey, Vinnie, you might be asking, if I can't eat sugar and grains, what's left?

Everything else.

You know how you've been avoiding steak and cheese to try and stay thin? Not any more. Ever pass by someone's house in the morning, smell bacon cooking and get pissed off because you've had Cheerios for a million days in a row? Guess what's back on your diet? Bacon.

What about those egg whites you were cooking in the Teflon pan? Are you crazy? Not only have you been giving up the yolk, the most nutritional part of the egg, you've been giving up the best tasting part. What a tragedy!

Fish, pork, steak, Italian sausage—all sausage for that matter—eat to your heart's content. And, from the plant world, what about all the delicious stuff you stayed away from because they were high-fat foods with lots of calories? Olives, avocados, coconuts. Enjoy!

You like heavy cream in your coffee? Dump it in!

And guess how much you can have of this stuff? As much as you want. When you start eating properly, when you rid yourself of those insulin swings, you'll lose the feeling of being a bottomless pit that can never be sated. You'll regulate the amount you eat naturally and you'll find yourself feeling full much quicker.

Don't believe me? Ask yourself this question. How many fat carnivores are there out in the wild? Answer: none.

You know what animals are fat?

Cows, pigs, domesticated creatures that are fed diets of grain. Hell, cows need four stomachs just to be able to digest the stuff. And while we're on the subject of domesticated creatures, look at dogs. Of all the different kinds of wild canines in the world—wolves, coyotes—it's only domesticated dogs that end up with a weight problem. Why? Because their kibble is full of corn, wheat, rice and other fillers.

So with all this talk of the 3 B's—bacon, beef and butter—you're probably thinking to yourself, what about cholesterol? Won't mine go through the roof? We've certainly been brainwashed to think so. It wasn't that long ago that people even knew what a cholesterol level was. And then, suddenly, we all became armchair experts, waxing poetic about good HDL and bad LDL. And how did we become such experts? The drug companies who make the statins gave us this info in sixty-second commercials.

But let's look at the facts from people who aren't trying to sell us something.

According to a new study conducted by The National Institutes of Health and published in the Annals of Internal Medicine, people following low-carb diets reduced their LDL (or bad cholesterol) in greater amounts than low-fat dieters. In fact, Dr. Gary Foster, PhD of Temple University's center for Obesity Research and Education, said that the notion that the low carb approach to weight loss was bad for the heart is "largely unfounded."

Here's what you have to understand—I don't have a dog in this race. I'm not trying to sell you something. Look at the cover of this book. Is it called *The Vinnie Diet*? No. I'm just a guy who's been helping people get fit for well into my third decade and I can tell you from experience that this works. And I'm not the only one saying this. There are scores of doctors and PhDs backing me up. One of my mottos is:

Quick to study, slow to change.

I don't follow fads, I follow results. Vidal Sassoon had an ad campaign back in the eighties, "If you don't look good, we don't look good." I have a different saying in my business. If you don't look good, I go broke. And, although I've never been broke, it doesn't look like fun. So it's in my best interest to keep my clients lean, mean and, most of all, healthy. Because another one of my mottos is:

Clients can't write me checks when they're dead.

I tell you all this because it works. I've seen it in action over and over, with celebrity clients, kids, executives, socialites, housewives, everyone. Doesn't matter who they are, every *body* works the same way and yours will, too.

Still not convinced? Try it for a few weeks. What do you have to lose except weight? If I'm wrong, which I'm not, you can always go back to your rice cakes and tofurkey and inedible Ezekiel bread. As for me, I'll be at Ruth's Chris with a New York strip and a side of creamed spinach.

After I teach my clients this new way of eating, they often decide to game the system. They see that they're losing pounds and inches quicker than they ever have in their lives and they get to thinking they can do it even faster if they remove a few more calories by only eating lean protein and cutting out the fats.

Egg whites only ... skinny lattes ... non-fat yogurt ... boiled chicken ...

This is a recipe for disaster, because when you cut the fat out of your diet, you also cut out the very thing that keeps you sated and gives you energy.

You don't need to game the system.

We've been conditioned to think that diets are supposed to make us suffer, but you don't need to suffer. As a matter of fact, if you're suffering, you're doing something wrong.

Look, it's really this simple: if you're always hungry you won't lose weight long term. Forget counting calories, forget watching your portion size, forget trying to eat low fat. Just do these two simple things.

STAY AWAY FROM SUGAR
and
STAY AWAY FROM GRAINS

Will this change of lifestyle be completely painless? Mostly, with one exception. A couple days after you begin, you might feel a little lethargic. Don't let this discourage you. It's just your body naturally transitioning from the sugar spike roller coaster it's been on for years to the healthy way it was meant to function. Within a day or so, that fatigue will go away and you'll find yourself with more energy than you've had since childhood. And how will this amazing thing happen?

One word.

Remapping.

Chapter Six
REMAPPING

I'VE ALWAYS BEEN a fan of motorcycles. They're great for commuting and saving on gas but, let's be honest, the real reason I like them is that they're fun. And you know where they're really fun? On a racetrack, where you can open them up full tilt.

My favorite track is Willow Springs on the way to the Mojave Desert in California. At certain times, the track is open to the public as long as you have the right gear.

The first time I went there, I saw these guys working on laptops that were plugged into their bikes.

"What are you guys doing?" I asked.

"Remapping the system," one of them said.

I'd never heard that term before.

They explained that a combination of state and federal laws restricts the way that bikes can perform on public roads, but the racetrack is the Wild West. No restrictions there. Which is why they were using their laptops to reprogram the computers in their bikes, allowing them to burn more fuel and go faster. By removing these restrictions, they were unleashing their bikes to do what they had been created to do—roar down the track like mechanized beasts.

They called the process "remapping."

I realized that this is exactly what I do every day with my clients. They usually come to me after trying to get fit by following one crazy diet after another, not realizing that those diets have been restricting their potential. They've cut back on their fuel, which left their metabolic engines sputtering along instead of becoming the speedy machines they were designed to be.

By simply changing the way they ate, I improved my client's metabolism, taste buds, energy and hunger. It helped them and now it's going to help you.

Once you start eating this way, your metabolism will change from a flame that flickered in the breeze into a roaring fire. Remember those calories that you used to count religiously, trying to keep the number as low as possible? Not any more. They'll now be consumed in that newly remapped metabolic furnace.

You know what I hate about a lot people in the health and fitness industry? They forget that they're dealing with humans. Just because some study or test was done in a controlled environment doesn't mean that you live in a controlled environment. We live in the real world and you know what's in that world?

Red velvet cake.

Spumoni ice cream.

Cannolis.

And, yes, even crullers.

We live in a world filled with delicious things and there are people who have to sell those things in order to make a living. What, you want them to go broke? How cruel are you? Look, I've just introduced you to a new and better way of eating but that doesn't mean you can't ever cheat a little. In fact, I want you to cheat so that you won't feel like you're missing out on anything.

Let's say there's something you really don't like to eat. For me, that would be cantaloupe. Don't ask me why. I like all the other melons, even cantaloupe's evil cousin, the honeydew. But if you told me I could never have cantaloupe again, suddenly I'd be dreaming about eating it.

Bottom line, we want what we can't have.

You may notice the four treats I mentioned—cake, ice cream, cannolis and crullers—have sugar or wheat in them and you might be thinking to yourself "isn't that stuff forbidden?" I'll tell you what I tell my clients when they ask me things like that.

It doesn't matter what you eat between Christmas and New Years, it only matters what you eat between New Years and Christmas.

I don't want to live in a world where I can't ever enjoy a red velvet cake or spumoni or cannolis or even a cruller, and I don't expect you to live in a world like that, either. Just don't do it every day. Make a treat out of it, not a habit. Remember back when treats used to be just that—treats? Something you enjoyed rarely enough that, when you had it, you called it a "real treat"?

So treat yourself on occasion. And don't worry. We remapped your metabolism into a roaring furnace, remember? You'll burn up the occasional doughnut or slice of pie quicker than a sheet of paper in a fireplace.

Let's talk taste buds.

Before you started eating like this, sugar overwhelmed everything. It was like a tsunami that drowned out every other flavor. But get ready for a surprise. You're about to discover a whole new world of taste.

You won't believe how delicious meats and cheeses will seem once their true flavors aren't camouflaged by a lifetime of sugar. And when you have something with natural sugar in it, like a piece of fruit, you're going to swear it was dunked in honey. It's time to enjoy food the way you were born to.

And you're not just going to remap your metabolism and taste buds, you'll also be remapping your energy. Remember how the motorcycle went faster once it started burning more fuel? So will you.

Once the sugar monkey is off your back, you're going to find that the gravitational pull that your couch once had will be gone. You might even, for the first time, want to exercise. Why? Because your body is finally releasing its fat stores and burning them as fuel. It's a two-for-one-special. You'll be feeling great and getting thinner at the same time.

And you won't be hungry, either.

When you have fat back in your diet, you'll feel full again, so you won't constantly want to graze like a cow. Even better, you don't have to keep feeding your sugar crashes with more sugar. Your appetite will return to the way it's supposed to be.

I'm in a storytelling mood, so let me tell you a story about a kid I trained. Let's call him Kevin, because that's his name.

I'd known Kevin since he was seven years old because his mom was a client of mine. Every year, I watched as he got heavier until he finally topped the scales at a whopping two hundred and thirty five pounds. At twelve years old, his mom sent him, for the third time, to an overpriced "fat camp" where a lot of celebrities shipped their kids.

When Kevin came back from camp that summer, I noticed something. Not only did he not lose any weight, I could have sworn that he'd gained some. How is this possible, I wondered. At the very least, if they were restricting the kid's diets, he'd have to lose something.

That's when Kevin explained the "two-suitcase method."

"One suitcase is filled with clothes," he told me. "The other is filled with candy." He went on to say that it didn't matter what you brought with you because, just like prisoners using cigarettes as currency, the kids at the camp traded their sweets among themselves to get exactly the kind they wanted. You'd think any decent fat camp would put a stop to this but, apparently, they were more interested in their "accounts receivable".

Believe it or not, that wasn't the thing that made my blood boil.

He showed me a picture. It was a black and white photo of him, shirtless with his large belly hanging over his shorts, standing in front of a concrete wall, holding a sign that said his name, the date and his weight. He looked like a convict. And the look on his face almost brought tears to my eyes. I asked him who was around when that picture was taken.

"Every other kid at camp," he replied. "It's the thing we dreaded most. Knowing we'd have to stand almost naked in front of everyone."

I saw red. I knew what I had to do.

Right then and there, Kevin became my next client. We started to ease into a workout program. Even something as basic as walking around the block was a chore for him. We counted his jump ropes—not in minutes, which is the way most people do it, but in the number of times he was able to complete a single jump. The first day, he couldn't get past ten.

Along with exercise, we started to talk about diet.

I couldn't tell him what to do until I knew what he was already doing. I needed to know what skeletons he kept in the closet before we cleaned it out. It turned out to be exactly as I thought. Pancake breakfasts, mid-morning bag of chips followed by a candy lunch. More junk food after school. He usually had a healthy dinner, because that was provided for him by his mom, but it was followed by more snacking while he did his homework at night.

It's amazing what the human body can endure.

Even though Kevin's mom believed in healthy eating, she couldn't control what he ate during the day when she was at work or when he was hidden away in his bedroom at night. I thought I was going to have a hard time convincing Kevin to change his ways, but the teasing had taken a toll on him and he was all ears. He wanted to do the right thing.

He cleaned up his diet immediately, dumping the carbs and sugar. Breakfast became bacon and eggs. Lunch became vegetables and fruit, along with cheese and cold cuts. Dinner remained the same—poultry, fish or beef, along with a small amount of rice or pasta. Snacks? Forget about it. Kevin was determined to beat this fat.

But something strange happened.

After seven weeks of exercising and eating properly, Kevin barely lost a pound. It was, as Vizzini says in *The Princess Bride*, "Inconceivable!"

We went over it again and again. I interrogated the kid, trying to break him down. I couldn't accept that I was failing or, even worse, that he was failing. Was I being lied to? Was he sneaking food? He swore he wasn't. I believed him. So what was it?

I found out when, days later, Kevin walked in while I was on the phone with another client. He heard me tell her how detrimental soft drinks were to her weight loss.

"Soft drinks are not your friend," I said. "They're nothing but liquid fat."

As soon as I hung up, Kevin said, "You never told me I couldn't have Coke."

I turned to him, surprised. "How many Cokes do you drink?"

He shrugged. "I don't know. Six or eight."

"Every day?"

"Yeah! I love them. I even have one with breakfast."

"Why didn't you tell me this before?" I asked.

"I didn't think it mattered," he replied. "You only asked me what I was *eating*."

I would love to say this was "kid logic" but you'd be surprised how many adults think this way, too.

So I spent the next week or so weaning Kevin off the liquid demon. The weight started flying off. His energy improved so much that, when I showed up, he would already be lathered in sweat from a twenty-minute jump rope session, ready to begin his real workout. It was hard to believe this was the same kid that I used to have to drag off the couch in a semi-coma.

One year later, he'd dropped a hundred and ten pounds and was a lean, muscular machine, filled with confidence and energy. He felt great, looked great and never looked back. Now in his mid-20's, Kevin has continued to eat properly and keep up his routine. He's married, employed and happy.

So what goes hand in hand with proper eating?

We all know the answer to that. Exercise. But we don't get enough of it in today's society. Know why?

Because our brains are killing our bodies.

Things are so convenient now that we hardly have to do anything physical any more.

Case in point: gyms that have valet parking. That's right. The people that own the place want you to avoid having to walk from the parking lot to the gym where you're going to get on a treadmill and, you guessed it, walk.

Crazy, right?

Hell, one gym I belonged to had an elevator from the first floor to the second, where you stepped off to find yourself facing a Stairmaster. That's right. They whisked you up a flight of stairs to get you to a machine designed to make you walk up a pretend flight of stairs.

And for those people who think stairs are too challenging, we've figured out a way to simplify sidewalks. Many airports now have moving sidewalks, so that you can go forward without ever being burdened by something as strenuous as taking a step. Vegas has them, too, but did you ever notice that the moving sidewalks only bring people into the casinos? If you want to leave, you have to exit the "hard" way.

You know, by foot.

What about dating? That used to take at least some effort.

Back in the eighties, if you wanted to get laid, you'd have to take a shower, comb your hair, put on some decent clothes and go to a bar or some place where you could meet the opposite sex. Nowadays, you can sit at your desk in your cruddy-ass underwear with a king-sized bag of chips and visit internet dating services without ever getting out of your chair. Hell, half the time you can get your date to show up at your door. And don't worry if you didn't bother to go out and pick up some wine—there's an internet service for that, too.

People try to excuse this with a simple word. "Convenience."

I have another simple word to describe it. "Laziness."

The easiest way to do something is not always the best, but we keep looking for the quick fix, and that even extends to parenting.

Recently, I started using a new term: Glow Kids. You've seen them. They're easy to spot because they're all lit up by a fluorescent blue hue from their handheld devices. You see kids all the time standing in line texting, sitting in restaurants with earbuds in their ears, lounging at home fiddling with apps. Whatever happened to talking, to communication? But Vinnie, you say, this is the new way people communicate. Get with the program!

Believe me. I get it.

But let me remind you how kids used to communicate. Shouting at each other while riding their bikes around town together. Running through the neighborhood, creating new games that made no sense to anyone but them. Hell, when I was a kid, I'd leave the house with a baseball, basketball and football because I was never sure what game we were going to end up playing.

In other words, we were moving. We were active. Not just sitting there, passive, pecking away at a piece of glass like a bird in a jar.

When I was in elementary school back in the swamps of Louisiana, I had a teacher who told us that she'd read an interesting article. It said that, one day, our brains would be the only thing we'd need to use and that our bodies wouldn't be necessary any more. My third grade mind imagined this as a bunch of heads without bodies sitting on tables. I never thought it would end up the other way around—a head sitting on top of a giant useless blob of a body.

But that's what we're creating today.

Back in the seventies, there were no TV commercials for fitness equipment, running shoes, diets or weight loss pills. We had commercials for terrible stuff like cigarettes and hard liquor, yet we were thinner and healthier as a nation because we moved more. We did it naturally as part of our daily living, not because we were told to do it. In fact, the only time exercise was mentioned on TV was when you heard things in an ad like, "I'd walk a mile for a Camel." Ironic, huh?

So that's the problem. What's the solution?

Simple. If we don't get our exercise naturally any more, we need to get it another way. I'm going to show you how. And I'm going to make it fun. This is a crusade for me. A passion. Exercise changed my life—and I mean that literally.

Exercise literally changed my life.

Let me tell you how.

Part Two

EXERCISE TO WIN

Chapter Seven
JACK LALANNE SAVED MY LIFE

WHEN I WAS six years old, I had a blockage in my ears that left me legally deaf. Fortunately, surgery corrected it. Unfortunately, this happened when I was learning to speak, so I had a terrible speech impediment. You know how deaf people sound when they talk?

That's how I talked.

At the time, I was living in Donaldsonville, a small southern town in Louisiana. It was a combination of Mayberry and that backward town where they wouldn't let you dance in *Footloose*. My parents were both public school teachers. I've never seen two people work harder to educate kids in my life. When I'm home, folks still come up to me and tell me what my parents meant to them. But, because they spent their whole lives working in the public school system, they knew firsthand how much it sucked, which is why they were determined that their kids go to private school. In Louisiana, most private schools have some sort of affiliation with a religion.

I went to Catholic school.

It was hell.

From the time I stepped on the bus until the time I got home, kids ridiculed me because of the way I talked. Even worse, I ended up repeating the second grade. After I finished it the first time, the nuns got together and told my parents I should stay back again because my math and reading skills were weak—even though I had passing grades.

This caused huge fights in my house, the only time I've ever seen my parents argue. My father thought that the stigma of repeating a grade far outweighed any extra benefit I might get. My mother disagreed. She thought that it wouldn't hurt me to mature a little.

Because I come from an Italian family, my mother won.

So I repeated the second grade, which only made the abuse worse. The kids teased me relentlessly. They called me "Vinna" because that's how I pronounced my name.

Even the nuns mocked me.

I'd try to participate in class and, as soon as I spoke in my Marlee Matlin style, they'd tell me to "get the grits out of your mouth" which only let the other kids know that I was fair game.

You think I'm exaggerating, but these nuns were no angels. Their favorite sport was coming up with new ways to torture kids and I was a favorite target. One of the reasons I didn't want to repeat second grade was because they had so much fun abusing me the first time around.

Here's an example. I was called to the front of the class for "deliberate disobedience." The nun told me to roll my pants up above my knees. While I was doing that, she walked over to her desk and pulled out a brown paper bag. She walked back to me, reached a hand into the bag and retrieved a fistful of uncooked Mahatma rice, which she sprinkled on the hardwood floor.

"Now kneel in it," she said.

I wasn't sure I'd heard right. "But there's rice—"

"Now."

There was a gasp from the classroom. I put my hands on the floor to ease my bare knees onto the hard kernels of rice. As soon as they touched, I could feel puncture wounds, so I immediately shot to my feet.

"You still want to disobey me?" she shouted.

"No, but—"

"Get on your knees now!"

I did. Even though I was in incredible pain, I decided that I wasn't going to let her beat me. I was just going to take it. And I was able to, until she walked up to me holding two paperback bibles.

"Hold your hands out," she said.

I did. She placed a bible in each hand to add to the weight driving my knees into the rice.

"If you drop either of these," she continued, "you'll be showing disrespect to Jesus and your time's going to start over."

But you never said how much time I had to begin with, I thought, so how can it start over? Luckily, I didn't say that. My hands quivered as I tried to hold as still as possible. Any movement made the rice dig deeper. From behind me, I heard a girl crying. Her name was Penny. I glanced at her and saw that she was looking at the two puddles of blood that had formed on the floor beneath my knees.

Finally, the nun turned to me and said, "Get up. You disgust me. Your punishment's over. Take a seat."

I did as I was told.

Later, when my mom asked me how I cut both of my knees, I told her I got hurt on the playground.

By the way, you want to know what I did to deserve such a punishment? During class, there was some construction going on outside. The nun had warned us to pay attention to her and not look out the window. Just then, there was a loud bang out on the construction site. The whole class, startled, looked over, then quickly turned back.

I wasn't quick enough.

I got the rice treatment because I'd looked out the window a second too long.

But it wasn't just the nuns who made my life hell. The other kids in school used to start fights with me as they mocked the way I spoke. One kid would kneel behind me while another pushed me backward, knocking me to the ground. I'd fight back and then more would pile on.

The bus was no better.

I rode with the public school kids, which meant there was a whole new crop of students to beat on me. One day, a couple of them got off a stop early just to kick my ass before walking home. Every day I'd go home with scrapes and bruises and tell my concerned mother that I'd fallen down in the playground.

This went on for years. There was no safe place to hide from the constant torment. I was in hell. I wished I was dead. Or a superhero. How great would it be to be able to fight back and protect myself? Unfortunately, even though I was only nine, I knew superheros were just cartoon characters.

There was no hope.

I tried to escape my life by watching Wide World of Sports on TV. I don't know if you remember it, but you could always see athletic people in exotic locations all around the globe. Over the course of an hour, you'd go from a motorcycle race on the Isle of Mann to a ski jumping competition in Kitzbuhel.

You're probably thinking the same thing I was thinking. Where the hell is Kitzbuhel? Answer: Austria.

I really wanted to go there. It looked so clean and the people seemed nice. I was in such a bad mental state that I thought a place that housed a Nazi death camp during WWII was better than where I was living.

And then, a miracle happened.

I was getting ready to turn off the TV after watching Wide World of Sports when a new show came on featuring a very muscled guy doing exercises. His name was Jack Lalanne. He seemed like a God and I wondered how he got to look like that. That's when my nine-year old brain put it together. Weight lifting.

For the first time, I realized that lifting weights up and down could lead to putting on muscle. And if you did it enough, you could maybe end up looking like Jack Lalanne.

Who needed cartoon superheroes? He was the real deal!

I wanted to start lifting weights. Unfortunately, I didn't have any. But what I did have was a hollowed out piece of metal pipe and a couple of bricks—the kind with the holes in the center. I'd slide the bricks onto each end of the pipe and lift it up and down. Which kind of worked, except the bricks would slide down the pipe and rip up my hands.

I didn't care. I did it anyway.

One day, my Uncle Frank asked me what happened to my hands. I told him about my gym in the backyard. He wanted to see it, so I took him out and demonstrated my lifting technique, promptly cutting my hands again.

"You really want to do this?" he asked.

I told him I wanted to be like Jack Lalanne. He said he knew someone better than Jack Lalanne, which I knew was bullshit because there wasn't anyone in the world better than Jack Lalanne.

Except there was.

Joe Bonadona.

This guy made Jack look like a wimp. His pecs were like Honeybaked hams. His biceps reminded me of oversized pythons. He had quads like sequoias, and a stomach that looked like it was carved out of marble by Michelangelo. My Uncle introduced us. Joe shook my hand in his giant fist and said, "Hello, Vinnie."

Not "Vinna." Vinnie.

For the first time in as long as I could remember, I met someone who didn't mock me. From that moment on, I didn't care
what anyone said, I was going to be like that guy.

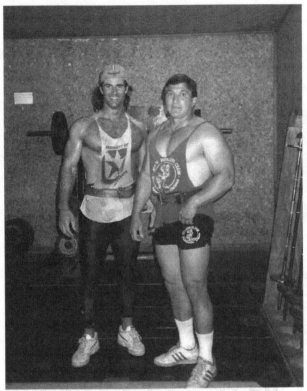

Me (years later, in my 20's) and Joe Bonadona at his health club.

He had a gym. It was about fifteen by fifteen, with walls made
of cinderblock and a tin roof. The equipment was made by a local
welder. The benches didn't have any upholstery—the seats were
raw wood. Instead of having pull-down machines, he had pullies
hanging from the rafters threaded with a rope tied to a t-bar that he
hung weights on. In the summer, if it was a hundred degrees outside, it was a hundred and thirty inside.

It was heaven.

Joe didn't allow many people to work out there. Aside from Joe, there was this other buff guy named Charlee. He had a great tan and long brown hair that hung halfway down his back. He looked like he belonged on the cover of a Harlequin romance novel, if the guys on those covers could kick your ass.

Then there was a black guy named Batiste, although everyone called him Bat. He was always quiet. He eventually moved to Ohio and did really well in body building competitions.

Finally, there was Joe's younger brother, Meatball. That's right, Meatball Bonadona. Meat was in pretty good shape, but he wasn't all that serious about working out. If the other guys spent four hours in the gym, he was in and out in an hour, and most of that time was spent cracking jokes. I liked him a lot.

And then there was me.

Joe had one rule I had to follow if I wanted to work out in his place. "I want you here five days a week," he told me. "If you miss a day, don't come back."

Looking back on it, Joe probably thought that a kid my age would never stick to the program and I'd be out of there in a couple of weeks, tops. What he didn't realize was that I was at such a low point that I was literally ready to hang myself.

It was my only shot.

So Joe told me not to miss a day and I never did. In fact, there were days I'd go to school with a fever because it was within walking distance of the gym and I needed the school bus to get me close to it, rain or shine, sickness or health. Those four cinderblock walls gave me hope for a better future.

As soon as I started pumping iron, my body changed quickly. In fact, adults used to tell me, "Be careful, because as soon as you stop working out, those muscles are going to turn to fat." But I knew that would never happen because I knew that I would never stop working out.

When I was eleven, Joe decided to take me from Donaldsonville, my small town in the Bayou, to Gonzalez, which had the first real gym I'd ever seen. He told me to bench press two-hundred pounds because he wanted to prove to the gym owner that he was training an eleven-year-old who could bench such a crazy amount of weight. But I didn't bench press two-hundred pounds that day.

I benched two-ten.

The reason was simple. I was used to the bench press at Joe's gym, which didn't have any foam padding on it. It was just raw oak, which used to stain the back of my t-shirts with blood when the wood cut into my skin. But that bench at the fancy gym was so comfortable that I was able to do another ten pounds easy.

The adults in the place were amazed. And supportive. It was a good feeling. Soon, the kids at school started to respect me and the teasing stopped.

Except that's not true …

The kids didn't respect or like me any more than they did before and the teasing got even worse. The only difference was that, now, the kids started coming at me in larger groups. So instead of fighting a kid here and there, I found myself fighting three or more kids at a time. And, of course, the school considered me the problem. Once you get that label, it never goes away.

This all culminated at the end of sixth grade, when a record five kids tried to beat the shit out of me. But I'd gotten pretty good at fighting by then and I ended up kicking the shit out of them. The only thing I suffered was a ripped t-shirt. But I knew I wasn't going to get away with it that easy. The coach, Lou Latino—and, no, I'm not making that up—saw the fight and took me to the office. On the way, we had a curious conversation.

"Do you know that there's actually a legal way to kick kid's asses and have people applaud you for it?" he asked.

"No," I said, but I was certainly interested in hearing more.

"Did you get held back a few years ago?"

I nodded. "Yeah." I braced myself, afraid he was getting ready to tease me. But he didn't say anything else. He just dropped me off at the office and they sent me home.

The next day, the coach called my house and told my parents that the JV football team was made up of eighth and ninth graders, although only the ninth graders really played. The eighth graders were basically blocking dummies.

My parents wondered what this had to do with me, because I was only in sixth grade. The coach explained that he did some checking and, because I was held back a year, I was a year older than the other students in my grade and, insurance wise, I would be eligible to join the JV team in my seventh grade year—something that had never happened in the history of the school.

So I joined.

The JV team got the hand-me-down crappy equipment that was dumped by the varsity team. The ninth graders got first pick. Then the eighth graders got what was left. Being the only seventh grader, I got the scraps that no one wanted. My helmet was made for high school kids, who were the size of adults. My head banged around inside it like a sneaker in a dryer.

Didn't matter. I didn't care.

We started practice and it turned out that I didn't know a damn thing. In fact, the main piece of coaching I got when I was playing defense was "hit the guy with the ball." Fair enough. I could do that. And I did it—a lot.

And then something miraculous happened. They posted the starting line up for the first game and I was on it. It was all ninth graders, a couple eighth graders and me.

Parents went batshit. They were furious that some of their kids got passed over so a seventh grader could play. But Lou Latino had my back. He told the parents that I earned my position and their kids didn't. It was that simple. Some parents grumbled that Lou was showing favoritism to a fellow goombah. "The dago's got the other dago's back."

Lou didn't give a shit. I was on the team.

Finally, it was time for the pep rally before the first game of the season. The bleachers in the gym were filled with excited, cheering students. One by one, every one of the ninth graders on the starting line-up was introduced and they were met with cheers and applause. Then the couple eighth graders who were on the team. They also got cheers and applause.

And then, finally, me.

Now, you have to understand, everyone at the school hated me. Hated me. I had spent my entire life tortured by these kids. So when I walked out onto the court for them to announce my name, I was prepared for boo's and catcalls. Instead, something completely unexpected happened.

The seventh graders cheered and gave me a standing ovation, which then prompted the eighth graders to do the same, followed by the ninth graders. Pretty soon, everyone in the school was standing and cheering me. And I stared at them and thought, *but they hate me. Why are they doing this?*

In retrospect, all these years later, I realize why.

It was because, for the first time, the seventh graders were being represented on the team and they loved it. It wasn't so much about me, it was about what I meant for them. And when they went crazy, everyone else in the school followed suit. In a weird sort of way, they were cheering for themselves.

The upshot of this was that, for the first time, they stopped picking on me. Now, if this was a movie like *Rudy*, this would be the last scene and you would leave the theater with your heart leaping and your eyes filled with tears. In reality, I got kicked out of the first game because, after one of the opposing players cheap-shotted me, I took off my oversized helmet and started beating the shit out of him with it. So ... not exactly the rousing climax of *Rudy*. But I'd done enough good things in the game up until that point that the coaches let me keep my starting position.

Four games into the season, another miracle happened.

It was almost halftime and we were way ahead. We were trying to put one more TD on the board before the half, and that's when I shattered my femur after a particularly aggressive tackle. Broke it so badly that, as they carried me off the field, my foot was facing backward. The doctor said that the bone had been broken in so many places that it looked like powder.

When I woke from surgery, I discovered that they'd placed me in a full body cast, all the way up to my armpits. I was immobilized. For eight weeks. And you know what happened while I laid in bed at home?

Girls from school came by to visit and hang out. The local priest stopped by on Sunday to give me communion. The hamburger joint sent hamburgers and a malt. Incredibly, I became one of the most popular guys in school by not being in school. I went from outcast to hero. I went from "Vinna" to "Vinnie." And it was all because, at the lowest point in my young life, a guy named Jack Lalanne showed me that, by changing my body, I could change myself and the way people reacted to me.

That's how I knew miracles could happen.

Our body is an amazing thing. It'll adapt to whatever we do. If we sit on the couch all day long, guess what? Our body will adapt and become large, soft and cushiony ... kind of like a couch. But let's say we spend that couch time on a bicycle. Chances are, over time, our bodies will become lean and sleek ... like a bicycle. Even though it seems like a miracle, it's really not. If you eat properly and exercise, you are going to get in shape. It's that simple. In fact, it's physiologically impossible to avoid!

Want to know one of the most common complaints I hear from new clients?

"Vinnie, I'm not even in good enough shape to get into shape!"

Don't worry about it. Since I'm your personal trainer now, let me ask you a few questions. Do you get out of breath from clicking the buttons on a remote control? Do you only stop eating because the bag of chips is empty and the pantry seems like too far to walk? Ever sleep on the couch because climbing the stairs to your bed looks like an expedition up the Matterhorn? If you answered yes to any (or all) of those questions, you know what you are. A classic couch potato.

Relax. You're not alone.

Everyone starts somewhere. And I have good news for you. If you're overweight, out of shape or don't exercise at all, you're going to discover that even a little bit of exercise will give you huge benefits. As your trainer, I have one simple goal for you right now.

I want you up off the couch and moving.

I'm not talking about running. I'm not talking about an hour on the elliptical. I just want to see you move a little. You'll be shocked to discover what a difference simply walking around the block a couple times a day is going to make to your overall health, endurance and flexibility.

At this stage, just getting started is the biggest obstacle you'll face. A lot of people like to walk with a friend or partner to give them the motivation they need to get out the door. But let's say you don't have a friend that fits into your schedule.

How about getting a friend that's always on your schedule?

If you're having trouble walking yourself, how about walking a dog? It's not unusual for people to get a pet to join them in their exercise. Even better, if you get one at the pound, you're not only saving a few dollars, you're saving a life—not to mention your health.

But let's say you're not ready for dog ownership. How about you borrow one?

Talk to friends and family or put up a sign around the neighborhood asking if anyone has a dog that needs exercise once a day. People will jump at the chance. Anything that gets you up and off that couch is going to start making you feel stronger and more alive. You'll feel better than you have in years and you'll start to think that it might be nice to fit into your clothes from a while ago. You know, that ones that are hidden away in the back of the closet.

Congratulations! You're no longer a Couch Potato!

It's time to take things to the next level. It's time to up the exercise program. Walking got us moving but, to really start seeing results, we have to move more. How do we go about doing that? We have to ride a bike in the open air, run across grassy fields, hike up tall mountains, or swim across wide lakes.

And where do we usually go to do all this outdoor activity?

In a small building called a health club.

Now I realize that many of us, me included, rely on health clubs to get our exercise. We don't all have access to mountains and clean lakes and, even if we do, we don't always have the time to visit those places. Some of us have local parks we could work out in but, if you don't have a permit to carry a concealed weapon, they may not be the safest choice.

So, somewhere along the line, after you've gotten up off the couch, you're probably going to find yourself in a gym. And, when you do, I just want to make sure you don't get screwed.

Chapter Eight
THE BIG SLEEP

SO YOU'VE FINALLY recovered from your New Year's Eve hangover and now it's time to make good on those resolutions to get fit, which means you're probably going to join a gym. But which one? Luigi's Gym and Pizza Emporium? Probably not. Instead, you'll find yourself at one of the mega gyms—Bally's, 24-Hour-Fitness, Equinox, just to name a few.

Here's what's going to happen.

You walk in to collect general info on the place. What's it look like, how much does it cost, what's the commitment? Your hopes are high and you're eager to get started on your road to health and sex appeal. The only problem is that you're an innocent. You think you've walked into a fitness center, but what you don't realize is that you've actually walked onto a used car lot, where they're selling memberships instead of clunkers.

You see that good-looking girl behind the counter? The blonde one with the killer smile who just welcomed you with open arms? She's stage one of their evil plan. In fact, you'd be hard pressed to find an unattractive male or female behind the desk of any gym. I also dare you to find one older than twenty five. Why?

Because youth and sex sells and they want you to look at that person and think *that could be me after a month at this gym.* That's their sole job, by the way, those people at the front door. They're the bait. But as soon as you say, "I'm interested in a gym membership," it's time for the switch.

They immediately page a sales rep.

The sales reps usually live in the little glass cubicles to the side of the front desk, so that as soon as the perky counter person pages them, they can all look out to size you up. They want to match you with the rep most likely to make you comfortable and get you to sign on the dotted line.

If you're a black guy, they're going to send out their black rep. If you're a woman, they're most likely going to send out a muscular dude who looks like a soap opera star. If you're a middle-aged guy, prepare for a hot chick.

Out one of them comes, smile on their face, hand outstretched. You're supposed to look at them and think *here's my partner on the road to fitness* but do you know what they really are?

Salespeople. Hardcore salespeople.

You might tell them you're looking at a few gyms in the area and they're going to tell you how great that is and promise to give you directions to the other gyms when you're done. Their goal is to find out your interests and make you think that they share those interests. They want you to believe that after you've done thirty minutes on the treadmill, you'll probably go out together and grab a Guinness.

If you like country music, they're from Nashville!

If you like fly fishing, they're going to Montana next weekend and think you should come!

Now that you're best buddies, they want to show you what they like about the gym. And here's where they differ from used car salesman—and I know about this because I was one in college. A used car salesman, while you're taking a test drive, will ask if you're interested in doing business that day.

This guy won't.

He's much smoother because, let's face it, he's got to sell you thin air. He doesn't have a car—hell, there's not even an actual object on the table. He's selling you fantasy, and to do it, he's got to engage in a little theater of the mind. The play he's performing today is called *The Fountain of Youth*.

So he takes you around, but he doesn't show you the fitness equipment—not yet—because that will remind you of exercise which seems like work. No, he's going to show you the spa, the whirlpool, the sauna. He's trying to paint a picture in your head that you're not actually joining a gym. What you're really joining is a country club and you and the beautiful people around you will soon be taking a soak together while sipping lime spritzers.

While this is happening, he's asking you questions.

He wants to know what sports you might have played in high school. If you played football, he's got some free-weights he wants to show you.

If you were a swimmer, just wait till you see their Olympic-sized pool!

If you played golf or any other sport that didn't require strength, there's some state-of-the-art aerobic equipment for you to check out.

If you were into dance, you have to see their yoga room with wall-to-wall floor mats and mirrors.

If you say you just knifed your entire family, they'll tell you about their advanced fencing program. What they're trying to sell you is your past. They want you to look at their gym as a fountain of youth that can send you back to the body you had when you had one.

Hang on. You smell that? That new car smell?

In the car business, that's called "the ether" and salesmen know that, once you smell it, you're in the mood to buy. You get woozy. In the gym, they've had you "smelling the ether" in the form of all the good-looking people around you, and you're getting woozy. But maybe you're not quite there yet, so it's time to pull out the big guns.

If you're a guy, the rep is going to walk you behind the hottest girl in the gym as she pumps up and down on the stair machine. And he's going to give you that look. You know the look. I don't even need to describe it. It's a mental high-five.

If you're a woman, they'll walk you past the free-weight area next to the guy with the glistening biceps and the tattoo that may or may not have come from prison. Either way, he's dangerous … and you like it.

In the car business, after they get you to smell the ether, they take you to "the booth." Once they've got you trapped there, they want you to sign on the dotted line before you realize that it's one of the biggest purchases you will ever make. How do they do this? They never talk about the big numbers—the purchase price and the insurance. Instead, they focus on the smaller numbers—the monthly payments and the "no money down." They speak in low, unthreatening tones. In New Orleans, we called it "the lullaby" and it was the process we used to "put you to sleep."

The gym wants to do the same thing.

But the difference between a car dealership and a gym is that, when you buy a car, at least you get to leave in it. You actually own a car. But when you buy a gym membership, all you really have is, well, nothing—except maybe that fly-fishing trip to Montana with your new best buddy and the girl on the Stairmaster.

Now remember, when you started, this guy was only going to show you around and give you some info on the place along with directions to the next gym for you to check out. But he's got to make the sale. Let's face it, he just spent the last forty-five minutes with you and he's got to convert this. He's got to put you to sleep.

He hasn't gotten you in the booth yet, so he needs to make that happen in the least threatening way possible. He walks you to the front of the gym as if he's going to point you in the direction of the other health clubs you said you wanted to check out. But, before he does, he miraculously remembers something.

"You know what …?" he asks.

At this point you're naturally wondering "What?"

He tells you he just wants to check something in the booth real quick, so he invites you in. He's mumbling to himself, "Did that end yesterday …?" He flips through some papers, glances at his watch and may even pick up the phone to talk to someone else, like Howie Mandel calling the shadowy banker on *Deal Or No Deal*. He's going to give a couple "uh-huh, uh-huh's" and then hang up. Guess what?

Great news!

You are so lucky he remembered to check on this, because there's an unbelievable membership deal that just expired—but don't worry. He can extend it. Not for everyone, of course, only for you. Why? Well, because you're fishing buddies and he really likes you.

That's lucky, you think, but you weren't looking to buy a membership just yet.

So you tell him that.

"But that's what's so perfect about this deal," he replies. It turns out that the first month is free. So, in essence, you're not really buying a membership at all. Now, yes, there is a two-year commitment after that first free month, but you can cancel at any time. If you don't like it—and he's sure you're gonna love it—you don't have to pay. It's risk free! Nothing in life is risk free and yet this is! And you know what?

He's not lying. It is risk free. You can cancel at any time.

But you won't.

Here's why. To give you this incredible deal, all he needs is a credit card. That seems reasonable, you think. So you give it to him. But now you're stuck, because once they have that card, they automatically charge it every month whether you use the place or not. Why is this so bad?

Because you forget you're paying for it.

And if you remember about it, you're still not going to cancel, because that would mean you're admitting defeat. That's you saying, "Screw my New Year's resolution and the promise of a great-looking, healthy body! I'm satisfied being the same old piece of crap I am right now just so I can save thirty bucks a month."

You won't do that.

At least, most people don't, and gyms count on this. It's how they make their money, and getting that credit card is the most important thing in the world to them. Don't believe me? Put it to the test.

Go into a gym, let them give you their whole song and dance and, when it comes time to pay for the membership, offer to pay in cash. They'll tell you they don't accept cash. What they don't tell you is the reason, which is that they don't want to keep asking you for money every month because, one day, you might say no.

They won't take that chance. They want to "put you to sleep" and forget about you.

You can explain to them that cash is actually legal tender. That it was printed by the federal government and is useable for all debt both public and private—it actually says so on the bill!

They'll tell you they're not set up to take cash. In fact, they'll tell you anything to get that credit card, because that's how they stay in business. This is as good a time as any to ask yourself a simple question.

What business is the fitness club actually in?

It's certainly not fitness.

They'll do as little as possible to continue to collect your money. In essence, they're in the collection business. Kind of like the mafia, but with less broken noses.

So you're almost ready to sign on the dotted line, but still a little hesitant. That's okay, because they're not done selling. They're going to sweeten the pot. Besides the free first month, the hot girl on the Stairmaster and a fishing trip to Montana with your new best buddy, the sales rep, they're going to give you five free sessions with a trainer. And not just any trainer. Your salesman is going to hook you up with the best one in the gym.

If you buy today, that is.

It's hard to see the downside in all this. Free sessions? You've heard these trainers cost hundreds per hour. And, the truth is, all that equipment is a little daunting. It would be helpful to have someone show it to you. But if you leave now and check out another gym, this one-of-a-kind extension being offered to you by your new best buddy is going to vanish along with your girlfriend, Susie Stairmaster, not to mention that fishing trip to Montana.

So do you sign?

Not yet. There are three things you can do to ensure that you get the best deal possible.

DO YOUR HOMEWORK

If you were buying a new car, you would never go to the dealership without knowing the true value of the one you want to trade in, as well as the invoice price of the one you want to purchase. In other words, you'd do your homework.

Treat a gym membership the same way.

Before you even visit, do a quick Google search and look for any special deals that the gym is currently running. Often, mega gyms will do cross-promotions with other companies, but the only way you'll know about this is to look for them beforehand.

For example, I got 30 percent off the membership fee for a gym I currently belong to by doing my homework and finding out that they had a cross promotion with CostCo. I was waiting for them to tell me about this when I went into the gym, but they never did. I had to tell them about it—and still they tried to pretend it didn't exist.

Like the Boy Scouts say: be prepared.

PAY FOR THE ENTIRE YEAR UP FRONT

Many people don't know that you can often get a huge discount off the membership fee by paying for the entire first year upfront—as much as 40 percent. In some cases, if you pay for two years up-front it's even cheaper. They don't tell you about this for three reasons.

The first is obvious. They don't like giving up any profits.

The second is psychological. Just like in the car business, they want to avoid scaring you away with big numbers, which means they're reluctant to tell you what an entire year will actually cost you.

The third is a little more devious. You can negotiate these deals so that they terminate after the first year, which means they can't continue to charge your credit card. As we already talked about, gyms hate to give that up.

Doesn't matter. All mega gyms offer this. Take advantage.

JOIN DURING THE LULL

You know when everybody wants to join a gym? In January, after the New Year, so they can fulfill those New Year's resolutions. Or just before summer, to get "bikini ready."

Sure, gyms will offer the "New You" deal or the "Red Hot Summer Special" during those periods, but you can get better deals if you're smart about when you join. It's simple supply and demand. Gyms need income all year and they're much more inclined to give you their best deals during their slowest months.

I'm looking at you, October.

So let's say you've found a gym you like and you've taken these three tips to get yourself the sweetest deal possible. Now you're officially a member of a mega gym. Did you make a mistake?

Maybe.

Here's what you've just bought—a promise. A promise for a new, healthier body. Only you can fulfill that promise and you do that by actually going to the gym and working out. But will you?

The statistics say no.

The majority of people who sign up at mega gyms never go back after the first few weeks. And it's a good thing, too. If everyone came to work out, the line at the elliptical machine would look like an Apple store the night before the new iPhone is released.

So how do you beat the odds? How do you get the most out of your gym membership? Two words.

Show up.

Chapter Nine
USE THE GYM,
DON'T LET IT USE YOU

SO YOU'VE JOINED a gym and you're determined to consistently show up and work out. You know what the gym thinks about this?

They're thrilled.

Now you can pay for more lessons with that trainer. You remember him, the best one in the place. The fact of the matter is, if you use the free trainer, learn the routines and come back regularly to work out, taking advantage of everything they have to offer, it will be the best money you've ever spent.

So let's say you're really going to do that. How do you get the most out of the gym? First of all, do you remember what gyms used to be like in the seventies? If you don't, go watch *Rocky* and then come back.

Okay, you're back. Adrian!!!

So now you know that gyms in the seventies were pretty much filled with free weights along with a pull up bar and couple jerry-rigged machines. Not to mention a chicken to help you work on your speed because, according to Mick, you gotta "eat lightning and crap thunder!" You know what? That stuff works.

Compare that to mega gyms now.

They're laid out like grocery stores. Go into any grocery store and what's the first thing you see? Crap. All the sugary, shitty, Nabisco-y products they want you to buy because they make the most money off them.

The gyms do the same thing.

Right by the register, you'll find a bunch of "health food" products, everything from protein bars to amino acid drinks. And they all have one thing in common: they're garbage. Look at the labels. Tons of sugar. Remember, you're in a health club. Hell, the name implies that you're in a club dedicated to making you healthy. But the place is sabotaging you as soon as you walk through the door just to make a buck.

And you know what product is the worst of the worst?

Look in the refrigerator next to the vitamin waters and the sport drinks. It's the thing that probably seems the most healthy, when, in fact, it's one of the most unhealthy things we consume and it can pack on the pounds quicker than anything else. What am I talking about?

Fruit juice.

Or, as I prefer to call it, a sugar bomb.

Fruit juice usually comes in two forms. Blended, which generally means they've added either sugar or other fruit juices to sweeten it, or all-natural. By the way, don't be fooled by the term "all-natural." Just because something is "natural" doesn't mean it's good for you.

Tornados are natural.

Think about what many of us do first thing in the morning to get our day started off on the right foot. We drink a glass of nutritious orange juice. In other words, a sugar bomb.

You'd be better off with the tornado.

Health clubs, like grocery stores, immediately bombard you with all this junk just to make a couple dollars. Ignore that stuff. Do yourself a favor and, on your way to the gym, stop by a convenience store and pick up a half pint of whole milk. It'll give you protein to build muscles and fat to sustain energy. What it won't give you is a mid-workout sugar crash.

So now you've pushed past the crap by the register. What do you see? In most mega gyms, probably row upon row of treadmills, ellipticals, stair climbers and other aerobic machines. Should you use them? Sure. Nothing wrong with them. You want to burn calories, go for it! They help build your aerobic capacity and they're also weight-bearing exercises which are great for your skeletal system—not to mention that women usually love what they do for their butts.

The problem is that most gyms place a twenty-minute time limit on the equipment, some even automatically power down the machine. Even though 24-Hour Fitness is open for twenty-four hours, it's only really busy a couple times a day, usually in the morning after all the mommies drop their kids off at school and in the early evening, after everyone gets out of work. And during that time, they don't want people waiting for machines. It's bad for business. But you know what else is bad?

Only doing twenty minutes of cardio.

Without getting too sciency, at twenty minutes, you've barely burned through your glycogen (the sugar in your blood), so you're not burning fat yet. And God help you if you drank that orange juice. It will take you forever to burn that sugar away. The benefit to your aerobic workout largely comes after those first twenty minutes, right when the gym wants you to stop. Bastards!

So what am I saying? Don't use the cardio machines?

Of course not.

Do it, but just don't go during rush hour if you can avoid it. And if you have to go during rush hour, do what I call the "Vinnie

Smorgasbord." Do your treadmill for twenty minutes, hop off it
and then hop right onto an elliptical machine or stair climber for
twenty minutes. Besides, doing one thing for an hour can get boring. Mix it up. Nike sold you those cross trainers, might as well use
them.

Okay, now you've burned some calories and you're ready to
put on muscle or get toned, which means you're headed to the
most intimidating part of the gym—the weights. People usually
avoid this area like the plague. Why is it so scary? Two reasons. The
equipment itself is a little nerve wracking but even more daunting
are the people using it.

They're generally muscular, which is unsettling if you aren't.
But that's not the worst part. It's the look on their faces as they sit
and stare at you when you enter. You think they're sizing you up,
like you accidentally wandered into a lion's den and they're looking
for fresh meat, waiting to pounce.

I have good news for you. They're not.

If you look at the people back in the aerobic area, you'll probably notice that they're all lost in their own worlds as they grind
away on their machines. That's just the nature of aerobic exercise.

Weight lifting is different.

When you lift weights, you have a few seconds of intense activity followed by a couple minutes of sitting there while your body
recharges before the next set. And what do you have to do in that
couple minutes?

Nothing.

So when someone new walks in, you naturally turn to them
because you have, literally, nothing else to do. They're not lions
lying in wait, looking for their next kill. They're just people trying
to catch their breath. Don't believe me? Try this. Next time you
walk into a weight room, look at one of them and wave. You know
what they'll do?

Wave back.

Trust me on this. If you need some help understanding the equipment, if you need someone to spot you while you lift, any of these people will be more than happy to lend a hand. Believe it or not, they tend to be far more friendly than the islands of solitude hammering away on the elliptical machines. Want to test that theory? During rush hour, go just one minute over on the stair climber and watch people scream for your head.

You won't find that in the weight room.

So what about the equipment? It sure looks intimidating. There seem to be a million different machines all doing a million different things. Not only that, for every exercise, there are usually several different brands of machine. You need to do a bench press? You might find a Nautilus, a Hoist and an Icarian. Why does the gym stock so many? Just to confuse you even more?

Not really. It's part of the sales pitch. They're trying to increase the odds that they have the particular brand that a prospective member might be familiar with. Don't let this throw you. You're looking at the forest. Focus on the tree, one machine at a time.

Remember that trainer you got free lessons from, the best one in the gym? Pluck him for information. If you didn't get any free lessons and you have no idea what you're doing, hiring one of those guys for a session or two will be money well spent. And if you can't do that, just ask around. Usually the other folks working out will be happy to help.

As useful as these machines are for building muscle and tone, there's something even better. If you've hit a plateau or your workout has gotten stale, maybe it's time to consider the next step up. Problem is, a lot of gyms have gotten rid of them. And many of the mega gyms, if they still have them, have shifted them into such a small area that they're hard to find. What am I talking about?

Free weights.

I know what you're thinking—please, God, don't make me use the free weights. If the machines are hard to figure out, and they only do one thing each, how am I ever going to figure out the damn free weights? There are infinite ways to use them, which means there are infinite ways to screw up.

I get it. They are more complicated. And for that reason it's best to move into them slowly. There's no shame in sticking with the machines. They can give you a great workout. But the men and women with the best bodies are going to be over by the free weights, because every single exercise you do with machines, you can do better with free weights. Why?

Your core.

First of all, what is your core? It's kind of like your lap. When you sit down, you have a lap. When you stand, it goes away. Or, if you don't like that analogy, try this one. It's like chicken nuggets. They exist in food form but try to point to one on a chicken.

The core is the same way.

We know it exists, we just don't really know where it is—like a g-spot. But now, everybody's obsessed with their core. We usually think of our core as our trunk, but it really refers to all of the support muscles that help the main muscles do their job. It used to be that you worked all those support muscles automatically. How?

Free weights.

Take a bicep curl. When you use a weight machine to work your bicep, it isolates only that muscle. But if you do the same thing with free weights while standing, you're not just working the bicep, but also your stomach, your total back, your hip flexors and your glutes, just to name a few.

In other words, your core.

Core, by the way, is a new term. We had to make it up because it used to be that you worked all those muscles automatically. Now you have to go to a Pilates teacher just to cover what you're lacking. We broke what was fixed. The bottom line is that free weights, used properly, are better for you than weight machines.

But try finding them in a mega gym.

Why? Liability. If used improperly, you can get hurt, which means lawsuits, which means money, something their bean counters don't like to part with. So how do you use them properly? If you still have some of those free training sessions left, I'd recommend that you do a session or two with the trainer and then try to do a session on your own. You know what you'll get out of that?

Questions. Good ones.

Write them down. Note the exercise you're confused about along with the weight you're using. Then schedule your next session with the trainer and get the answers.

Now I know what you're thinking. How much is this guy expecting me to do? I'm not looking to be a bodybuilder. I can't live in a gym. I have a life.

Of course you do. I know how busy you are. You work. You have to get the kids to their violin lessons and it's not like there's no traffic on the freeways nowadays. Which is why I'd love to be able to tell you that you can have ripped abs and buns of steel working out only ten minutes a day.

But I can't because it's not true.

Look, I promised not to lie to you because you've been lied to enough by unscrupulous magazines, infomercials, and ads that are all trying to sell you the idea that you can get the body of your dreams in no time flat. How do I know they're all bullshit?

Years ago, in my twenties, I was hired to star in an infomercial for a fitness product that promised to give you a rock hard body in just "minutes a day." They filmed me for over two days, showing my well-oiled muscles glistening as I used their machine. What they didn't show was that I had never even seen this machine before I got hired to do the commercial. And, as for their claim that you could have a body like I did back then in just "minutes a day"? It was absolutely true.

As long as you were talking about two hundred and forty minutes a day.

That's right. It took me four hours of intense weight lifting and aerobics, along with the perfect diet, in order to get the body that they promised their machine would give you in no time flat. They ran that ad for well over a year and it actually won infomercial awards.

That's right. In Hollywood, they even have awards for lying.

Which is why, as much as I'd love to promise you that you can have the body you want with no work and no time investment, I can't. I'd rather tell you the truth and have you accomplish something real, than lie to you and have you accomplish nothing. But first, let me ask you a question.

Why do you want to exercise?

Chapter Ten
WHY DO YOU WANT TO EXERCISE?

I'M NOT TRYING to be cute, it's an honest question.

We normally go out of our ways to avoid doing anything that requires effort. Case in point, back-up cameras in cars. Remember when you used to have to go through the trouble of actually turning around to see what's behind you? Not any more. You run over a kid today, you meant to. We'll do anything we can to avoid actual effort so, with that in mind, let me ask you again ... why do you want to exercise?

Here's what most people answer: "Because I want to lose weight."

That's fair. In fact, the entire exercise industry—including what I do—is built on selling you the idea that exercise will lead to a leaner you. But I promised to tell you the truth, so here it is.

Sweat does not equal fat loss.

If you take a pound of fat and wring it out, not one drop of sweat will come out. You can sweat your ass off but that won't get rid of your ass. To be clear, working out and burning calories certainly won't hurt your weight loss, but the single most important thing you can do to lose weight is to focus on your diet. As we talked about before, a proper diet—no sugar, no grains—is the most critical weapon in your weight-loss arsenal.

Want me to prove it?

Take a look at linemen in the NFL. These are huge guys. Want to know their average weight? Over three hundred pounds. Do you know how much time these guys put in the gym? Tons—which, by the way, is what they're lifting.

These guys aren't messing around with yoga and Pilates class. They're slinging steel. I'm talking about quarter of a ton squats and dead lifts. I'm talking about workouts so strenuous, just watching them do it makes you want to take a knee. Moving that much mass for hours on end burns a ton of calories.

But, Vinnie, you say, what about cardio? Sure, they're lifting weight, but do they run? That's where you really burn calories, right?

Sure, they run. Not only do they have off-season sprint programs put together by their team experts, they also have agility drills on top of loads of time on the spinner for general fitness. These guys burn massive amounts of calories in the gym—far more than you or I ever will.

And, yet, they're fat.

The reason? These guys, the linemen, intentionally eat to pack on the pounds.

Because diet is, by far, the most important factor
in weight loss and gain.

Why do they eat like this? Why do they want to gain so much weight? Survival. They know they're going to be slamming up against guys with as much or more weight than they have. In fact, the NFL has been quietly trying to get these guys to slim down to keep them healthy. Not that the NFL is some kind of kumbaya Florence Nightingale organization, they just want to protect their investment.

The point is, even though the calories burned during exercise will contribute to weight loss, you don't have to exercise to lose weight. You can lose all the weight you want through diet alone. In fact, my nephew wanted to test this theory. He didn't have a gym membership, never stepped on a treadmill and never lifted a barbell and yet he lost over sixty-five pounds strictly through diet. If he can do it, so can you.

Now, with that sobering fact in mind, let me ask you again:

Why do you want to exercise?

Remember, aerobic exercise is great for your cardiovascular system, not to mention your muscular and skeletal systems, but you don't have to do it to lose weight.

Anyone? Bueller? Bueller?

Let me take a crack at it. We need to exercise because, in order to achieve a maximum level of health and fitness, we have to move our bodies.

Did you just nod off?

Well, I did and I was actually the one doing the talking. Look, what I just said is the truth—in order to stay healthy, we have to exercise. But here's another, bigger truth: you probably don't care. I could write chapter after chapter explaining how exercise strengthens your heart and can help improve your longevity but, let's be honest, at the end of the day what most people care about is how they look.

We care about this so much, in fact, we'll pursue sex appeal even at the expense of our health. Case in point, men and women actually inject poison into their faces to get rid of wrinkles. We have no idea what the long-term effects of Botox are, but people do it anyway because they want to look great. I don't think Botox makes you attractive, by the way, unless you think looking perpetually startled is sexy.

Even though most people care more about their looks than about their health, I have some good news for you—exercise gives you both. It's a two-fer. Like I tell my clients:

> *If I can get you healthy by appealing to your vanity,*
> *I'm not above it.*

So how does exercise improve your looks if you don't really need to do it to drop weight? Let me ask you a question. What's the best-looking version of you? Is it the skinniest version?

Magazine ads want you to think so.

How many times do we have to see what I call "the super-model race" to see which sticks out farther, their cheek or hip bones? If you saw these women on the street, you'd think they were heroin addicts. When did we start using the aliens at the end of Close Encounters as the model for beauty? You know who thinks these emaciated women are sexy?

No one.

At least no one sane. If you're a woman and you finally made it to a size 0 but you have a saggy butt and loose skin on your arms due to muscle loss, is that what you were looking for? A body that looks like Willem Dafoe's face? If you're a guy and you hop on a scale and you're the lightest you've ever been in your adult life, but you just lost an arm wrestling match to a toddler, is that what you were looking for?

It's true that diet will help you lose weight, but losing weight is only one side of the coin. The other side—just as important—is putting on lean muscle mass. That's what turns Olive Oyl into Shakira and Shaggy into Channing Tatum, but you can't get there through diet alone. So let's talk exercise. How much do you need to do per week to see results?

Well, let's look at our options.

If we follow Tim Ferriss's plan in *The Four Hour Body*, we only have to invest four hours a month in the gym to get the body we want. That's pretty good! That's only one hour a week, or just over seven minutes a day. I'll take it!

But wait! Why settle for spending all that time in the gym when we could follow Jennifer Jolan's advice in *5-Second Flat Belly Secret*. My God, Jennifer is telling us that we can have a flat belly by working at it just five seconds at a time. That's way shorter than seven minutes!

Tim, you suck!

Not only that, but Jennifer promises we can get there without hard exercise and eating differently. We just have to use the palm of our hand to "literally 'burn' fat cells away." I've used the palm of my hand for many things, but never that!

Holy shit, let's do it!

By the way, her book sells on Amazon for $2.99. I'll make you a deal. Give me two dollars and I'll save you a buck by telling you not to buy it.

Here's the truth, and like most things that are true, you probably already knew it.

When it comes to exercise, you're going to get out of it
what you put into it.

Is one hour a day, three days a week enough time to see results? Sure is. Give me that and I can show you definite improvement. But you want to know what will give you even better results?

One hour a day, four days a week.

And guess what will give you even better results than that?

One hour a day, five days a week.

And it doesn't even have to be an hour a day. You could do a couple hours a day a couple times a week. You get out of it what you put into it. As I tell my clients, lean muscle mass ain't cheap and you can't buy it with money.

Exercise is a great leveler. It doesn't matter how rich you are, you can't just buy your way into a great body. You have to do the work. Lady Gaga has to grind her way through a workout just like the rest of us. I find that comforting. It's one of the few things in life where we're all on a level playing field.

But what about steroids, you ask? Aren't they a great short cut? Won't they make me bigger, stronger and give me that lean muscle mass?

Of course they will.

But there's a trade-off. A big one.

There are many kinds of steroids out there and, if used properly under a doctor's supervision, and at the right dosage, they're enormously helpful and can save lives. Often, they're employed to put lean muscle mass on patients who are wasting away. Guess who noticed that particular effect and said to themselves "I wonder ...?"

Yeah. Bodybuilders ... along with other athletes and coaches.

Instead of taking a carefully prescribed dose to treat an actual illness, these bodybuilders started injecting themselves with massive quantities of the stuff. Ten, twenty, even thirty times larger than the amounts used in medicine. And guess what they were delighted to discover?

It worked!

Still does. If you slam yourself with a ton of steroids, pump iron and eat protein, you are going to put on tons of muscle, guaranteed. The steroids artificially increase your testosterone, which is instrumental in causing the growth of lean muscle mass.

At a price.

Like the fabled blues players who wanted to be the best musicians in the world by going to the crossroads to make a deal with the devil, those athletes were making their own deal with the devil. Testosterone in such absurd quantities wreaks havoc with your endocrine system, which can have a bunch of terrible side effects.

Guys, do you like having zits and hair sprout across your entire body, while your ball sack shrinks to the size of a peanut? Not that a giant ball sack is the height of beauty.

Ladies, do you like having a penis-sized clitoris, along with a voice deeper than James Earl Jones? In fact, in the early eighties, the coach of an Olympic female volleyball team from one of the Eastern Bloc countries was asked why the voices of the women on his team were so manly. His reply, "We came to win, not sing."

And those are only some of the *cosmetic* side effects.

Let's not even talk about the real danger—the damage to your kidneys, liver and other vital organs. You can die from abusing these medications.

To summarize, here's the good news. Steroids work!

Here's the bad news. They will make your balls shrink, your clitoris grow and may end up killing you!

As I like to tell my clients:

Steroids can turn you into a great looking corpse.

So now that we've agreed to pass on the steroids, let's talk about what you can accomplish in a gym in an hour a day, three days a week, which, as your trainer, I think is a reasonable amount to ask you to do. Some days you might want to spend the whole hour doing cardio—elliptical, treadmill, the spinner (otherwise known as the stationary bike.) Other days, you might want to split it up and work in some weights.

The bottom line is, on an hour a day, three day a week workout, the most important thing you can do is vary your routine.

Let's talk weights. What exercises can you do that will give you the most bang for your buck in the shortest amount of time? By that I mean which exercises will work the most muscles at once?

First up—legs.

The three exercises that work the most leg muscles (including your butt) are: squats, lunges and leg press.

Before we go any further, I debated whether I should use some of those little illustrations to demonstrate how to do these exercises. You know the ones I'm talking about, the ones like this:

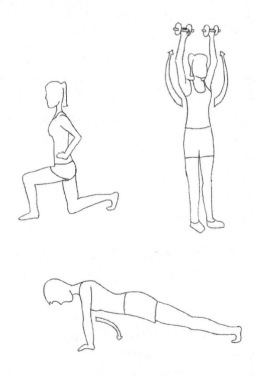

Do you like those? Me neither. If you're going to spend all that money to make a book, why hire a fifth-grader to do the illustrations? I hate those things. Know what I hate even more? Photos of the author demonstrating the technique with the gratuitous "Oh, I didn't know my bare abs were actually showing in this picture, but aren't they great?" shot. So I was trying to come up with a way that I didn't hate to show you how to do this stuff, and I finally found one. If you go to www.youtube.com/user/AngriestTrainer it'll take you to my YouTube channel where you can see videos of people demonstrating these techniques and many others. We're only going to skim the surface of these exercises here. If you want to learn about them in depth, check out the videos.

Okay, back to legs. Squats, lunges and leg press are the exercises you want to focus on. You can choose to do one, two or all three per session, depending on the amount of time you have.

How do you know how much weight to use for a given exercise? It's simple. If you've never lifted weight before, or it's been a long time, you pick an amount of weight that you can easily handle for up to fifteen repetitions over the course of no more than two sets. To be clear, a repetition (or rep) is the number of times you lift the weights in a row. When you're done, that's considered a set. Do this for a couple of weeks before you graduate to the kind of lifting you'll be doing from then on.

At this point, you want to pick an amount of weight that you can do for three sets of ten repetitions with some difficulty. Once you can easily do three sets of ten reps, increase the number of reps to eleven each set. Once you can easily do that, increase the number of reps to twelve. And once you can do three sets of twelve reps each, then it's time to move up in weight. How much more weight? Enough to make three sets of ten reps difficult once again.

Rinse and repeat.

Second category—upper body.

Just like with your legs, there are three exercises that give you
the best bang for your buck: bench press, shoulder press and lat
pulls. But unlike the three leg exercises, these hit different muscles,
which is why you should do all three whenever you're working
upper body.

Finally, abs.

Truth be told, your abs get worked a lot when you're doing
aerobic activity like running, cycling and elliptical, but it doesn't
hurt to throw in some sit-ups or a few sets on the gym's ab
machines when time permits.

This, by the way, brings me to another Vinnie-ism.

You want great abs, work on your diet.

Contrary to what the magazines would have you believe, the
only way to get washboard abs is to lose the fat around your
middle. You can do sit-ups and ab work around the clock and
never achieve what you're after because no matter how much
muscle you build on your stomach, you can't see it through fat.
And, just to clear up a common misconception, sit-ups don't help
you burn fat around your middle. In fact, you can't spot-lose fat in
any area solely through exercise. As I tell my clients, if you want to
spot-lose fat, get liposuction.

In case you're wondering, getting liposuction is a bad idea, just
like taking steroids. Want to know another bad idea? Colonics.
They're basically the same concept as liposuction. With liposuction,
you're paying someone to suck your fat out. With colonics, you're
paying someone to suck your crap out.

Think about that for a second.

There are people out there so desperate to lose weight that
they think having a hose shoved up their ass is a reasonable way to
accomplish this. And not just for them—for you, too. I've had
people try and convince me to let someone bury a hose up my

backside as if their lives depended on it. It's like a cult. You know why I've never done it? It's not natural. You know how I know that?

My ass didn't come with a spigot.

So, how might a typical one-hour a day, three day a week workout look?

Monday: Forty minutes of cardio. During the remaining twenty minutes, do all three upper body exercises and pick at least one of the leg exercises.

Wednesday: Forty-five to sixty minutes of aerobic activity. And don't forget the Vinnie Smorgasbord, where you use a variety of machines for shorter lengths of time. This is also a great day to do your ab work—some sit-ups or a set or two on an ab machine.

Friday: Just like Monday. Forty minutes of cardio, twenty minutes of weights. The only difference is that you're going to want to do at least two of the leg exercises, even at the expense of one or two of the upper body exercises.

By the way, if it takes you a few minutes more than an hour to get in your cardio time along with the weights, I got news for you—the world's not going to miss you. Take the extra few minutes. Just get it done. And remember, you can't follow a routine unless you actually get to the gym, so make getting there a priority, even if it's on a Saturday or Sunday. As I tell my clients:

Your body doesn't know it's the weekend.

Now, do you have to stick with the tyranny of my little schedule? Hell, no. Once you're there, mix it up. Make it a little different every time. Don't get stuck in a rut. Take advantage of the classes the gym has to offer. Pilates, yoga, aerobic dance, spinning—they're usually free with the membership or pretty cheap. Find one you like and do it. If you need motivation, let the teacher give you some.

You paid for all this thin air the gym sold you, so use it! Move your body! Don't be one of the eighty percent that wastes their hard earned cash. And don't let the gym push you around with their rules and regulations.

I was at a Bally's a few years ago, working out on a spinner. You know how when you work out hard, you sweat?

So do I.

After working out for a few hours, I was sweating. Really sweating. In fact, the floor was wet. So the gym manager comes up to me and tells me I need to mop the place when I'm done. I tell him I'm not the janitor. Shouldn't cleanup be part of my gym membership? He goes away.

Next day, same thing happens.

I'm spinning and sweating. Except, this time, when the manager comes up to me, he brings two musclehead trainers with him. Tells me to get off the equipment because I'm sweating too much. I see these guys and think, good, I'm about to get an upper body workout, too.

Back then, Bally's had a promotion where they said you'll "get in the best shape of your life!" Well, while this guy was telling me to get off the equipment, I notice a banner behind him that says exactly that: "Bally's—for the best shape of your life!"

I tell him, if I get off now, you're stopping me from getting in the best shape of my life, which would violate your agreement with me, which means I'll be back with an attorney and, by the time I'm done, "Bally's" will be renamed "Vinnie's" (a much better name for a gym, anyway, don't you think?)

He left and never bothered me again.

Get your workout. Don't let them push you around.

Now, eventually, you might find yourself enjoying all this physical activity and reaping the benefits of good health so much that you'll want to take it to the next level. Maybe you want to run a half marathon or your friend told you about a charity bicycle event and you've never ridden that far before. Can the trainer at the gym get you ready for this? Probably not. You need someone with a broader range of expertise—a *real* personal trainer.

If so, great! By all means, hire one. But, just like with health clubs, there's a lot of ways you can get screwed.

Chapter Eleven
TRAINERS ARE LIKE ASTRONAUTS

YOU EVER SEE the movie *The Right Stuff*? Great movie. It's about the history of the astronaut program. In the beginning, they took test pilots, duct-taped them into tin cans and shot them into space. They were like monkeys. In fact, they actually started with monkeys and worked up to these idiots.

No offense. To monkeys.

Let's take a second to imagine the conversation that led up to this.

Science guy: "Okay, Jimmy. Here's what we're gonna do. You see this gigantic bomb filled with enough highly explosive material to blow it all the way to space? Now, you see that little thing on the tip of the bomb? We call that a chair, Jimmy. You're gonna sit in it and then we're gonna light this thing on fire and see what happens."

Jimmy: "Okay."

Science guy: "Now stick with me. We think there's a fifty-fifty chance we can shoot you into outer space. But here's the problem."

Jimmy: "The fifty-fifty wasn't the problem?"

Science guy: "No. If we get lucky and you end up in space, we don't really know how to get you back. So you might just bounce along the outer atmosphere until you disintegrate. Sound good?"

Jimmy: "Okay."

So, that's how NASA started. But as the space program evolved, Jimmy wasn't good enough any more. We needed a different kind of cowboy. One with balls the size of Montana attached to a brain the size of, well, Montana.

Because we were getting fancy.

Now we wanted Jimmy to actually do stuff—like pilot the ship and walk on the moon. Astronauts had to become highly skilled.

Same with trainers.

In the sixties, a trainer was a guy in a gym with great pecs and biceps wearing a stained t-shirt with block lettering that simply said "TRAINER." We haven't improved much on the t-shirt, but the quality of trainer has come a long way.

Back then, trainers only had to know one thing—how to lift weights.

Jogging was non-existent. Since jogging was non-existent, so were marathons. Well, they existed, but they were left to runners, not joggers. Cycling? Say what? Competitive swimming? Forget it. The only time we even saw a swimmer was in the Olympics. And triathlons didn't even start as a sport until the late 1970s. So all a trainer had to know back then was how to do a bench press and a squat.

Compare that to now. Today's trainers are expected to be a combination of running coach, cycling coach, weight-lifting coach, nutritionist, stretching instructor, amateur orthopedist, motivational speaker and armchair psychologist.

In other words, not Jimmy.

So how do today's trainers acquire all these skills? By putting in the time.

At fifteen years old, I started teaching people over twice my age how to lift weights at Joe's Health Club. That's Joe as in Joe Bonadona. I was flying by the seat of my pants, kind of like Jimmy duct-taped to that rocket. And I loved it.

By the time I was eighteen, I got a scholarship to Tulane University, one of the foremost medical schools in the country. I knew I wanted to do one thing and one thing only.

Become a P.E. teacher.

Now, I know what you're thinking: "Vinnie, you sure set your sights high." But remember, I worked in a gym for many years for no money. My only pay was a key to the gym. All I cared about in life was how to get myself and other people fit.

At Tulane, where I went to college, in order to get a physical education degree, you had to jump through two hoops. First, you had to get your teaching credentials by being accepted into their secondary education program. Second, you had to take classes about the human body, which you could only get in their pre-med department.

That's how I ended up taking courses in biology, kinesiology, physiology and gross anatomy. The classes were difficult as hell, but I found learning how the human body functions fascinating. Still do.

As science and medicine advance, I'm right there trying to learn everything I can. After doing this for almost three decades, I think that I have the bare minimum of knowledge and practice that it takes to be considered an "expert."

But that's not the case with many so-called trainers today. Sure, there are a lot of good ones, even great ones. I'd like to say there are also a lot of shitty ones, but it's worse than that. A shitty trainer will take your money without helping you improve, which means all you'll lose is time and money. A worse than shitty trainer will get you hurt—sometimes permanently. So how are people like that able to call themselves trainers?

The same way dog walkers are able to call themselves dog walkers.

If someone wants to be a dog walker, they can literally wake up, pour a cup of coffee and utter the words "I think I want to be a dog walker" and they're in business. All they need is a clientele of dogs.

Same with trainers.

Anyone can claim to be a trainer.

In the early eighties, my training business was rolling right along down in New Orleans. I was one of the few trainers in the city or, to be honest, in the whole country. Jake, as in "Body By", had been doing his thing out in L.A. for a few years but I guess people were tired of writing about him and were looking for a different face, so I started getting some press. I even made it into an issue of SHAPE magazine. I wondered when the competition would come along.

What I didn't realize was that my competition was right under my nose.

Let's call this woman Emily. I guess I worked with her for two weeks, a total of six times. Emily was different from every other client I'd had up until that point. Most of my uptown socialites didn't care how they were losing weight. They just wanted to know that they could continue to eat shrimp remoulade and still fit into a size 2.

Not Emily!

She wanted to know how it worked, how the routines were laid out. She paid attention to sets and reps and wrote everything down. She even took me for coffee afterwards where she grilled me for details. She cared.

I loved her. It was like I had my first groupie.

But after exactly six hours of training her, she didn't schedule any more sessions and I couldn't get her on the phone. Within a month, I started hearing about a new trainer in town ...

I don't really need to tell you who it was, do I?

My old client, Emily, became a personal trainer just by taking a couple sessions and then calling herself a trainer. She had no degree, no certification, no anything.

Things haven't improved much since then. The only real difference is that, now, prospective trainers usually want to get some kind of certificate because most gyms require them for insurance reasons.

So where do you get one of these magical pieces of paper?

Well, you used to have to take a weekend course. In other words, these people covered in one weekend what it took me four years at a medical university to learn. But apparently, a weekend was too much of a time investment for a lot of people, so they made it even easier to get a certificate.

I mentioned this to my buddy, Scott. He didn't believe me. So he went on the internet and, within an hour and a half, became a certified fitness trainer with a certificate that would be accepted at any gym. Scott's day job? Attorney. Which means, when he hurts a client, he can now sue himself.

By the way, don't laugh. Scott could just as easily have become an ordained minister. Don't believe me? Google it. You'll find a hundred websites that tell you to fill out a form and pay a fee. Three days later, you'll be legally performing weddings.

You know what I call ministers like that? Frauds.

You know what I call personal trainers with these bullshit online degrees? You got it. Ministers.

How insane is it that you can get a certificate asking people to trust you with their bodies simply by spending a few minutes online? Who are these organizations handing out certificates to trainers like condoms at the free clinic?

Remember our dog walker? Well, one day, his dog walking business dried up, so he decided to open a training certification business. It's that easy ... and that corrupt.

Knowing all this, how do you find a personal trainer with legitimate credentials like an actual college degree in fitness?

Not by asking them.

Many trainers have figured out that prospective clients, especially in Beverly Hills, expect them to have a college diploma, so they'll lie and say they do. You need to make sure. Ask your potential trainer to physically show you their diploma. Anyone who actually graduated from a university should be happy, even proud, to prove they did. And if you're too shy to ask, call their university. They'll let you know.

This may seem like overkill, but it's your health we're talking about. People spend more time researching a pair of tennis shoes on the internet then they do making sure their trainer is qualified to keep them safe. Do it right.

So how do you figure out the best trainer for you?

In general, trainers who are not attached to a gym are usually better than trainers who are. Why? Two reasons.

First, money. Trainers at a gym have to split their fee with the gym, sometimes giving them as much as 50 to 70 percent. But if you're not attached to a gym, you don't have to pay that. So why would someone be affiliated with a gym?

Because they have to be.

Trainers attach themselves to gyms because they're not good enough to get clients on their own. Look, here's how I get clients. I train someone, they like what I'm doing for them, they tell a friend and then I get hired by that person.

But that's not how trainers in gyms get clients.

They work like ski instructors. Ski instructors use a "turn and burn" system. They realize that you're only going to be at the resort for a week, so they don't care about return business. The gym trainer also doesn't have to worry about return business because, chances are, you won't return after the first couple weeks—most members don't. Besides, they don't need you long-term because the gym will just throw them another client. Unlike personal trainers in business for themselves, the gym guys don't have to earn their clients through hard work and knowledge—they just have to be breathing.

The bar is ... low.

By the way, when I talk about gym trainers, I'm talking about the guys who work in mega gyms. The trainers who work in small, private gyms usually know what the hell they're talking about.

Want another story?

In the late nineties, I was working out at a mega gym. My grandfather was a janitor his whole life, which is why I have a soft spot for them. I respect them. The janitor at this place was named Jorge. He literally swabbed out the toilets. Every time I saw him, I said hi.

Nice guy. We were friendly. This went on for a year.

One day, while I was working out, I saw him on the fitness floor wearing a "TRAINER" t-shirt. I asked him what was going on. He said they told him they needed a Spanish-speaking trainer and then gave him the shirt. Those were his qualifications.

He could speak Spanish and wear a shirt.

Caveat emptor, which Wikipedia tells me means "buyer beware." So, buyer, let me tell you exactly what to beware of so that, just like with gym memberships, you don't get ripped off.

Chapter Twelve
BUYER BEWARE

SO YOU'RE IN the market for a trainer. Like a guy in a whorehouse, there are a lot of ways to get screwed—mostly by hiring amateurs. Here are some of the types you might encounter.

THE SOCCER MOM TRAINER

These are usually women who are looking to bring in some extra income to support their shoe shopping habit, because, let's face it, they can only get yelled at by their husbands so many times before they need to start making their own money. They have to figure out a way to do this and still be available at 3 p.m. to pick up their kids from school and then drop them off again at the soccer, or football, or baseball field. So they need to find work with flexible hours and good pay.

Manolo Blahniks ain't cheap.

By the way, this isn't their first job. Some of their other "careers" may include dog walker/groomer/sitter, working as an assistant in a pre-K and doing portrait or sports photography. Hell, I even knew one that tried to be a comedian.

None of these things are bad, necessarily. The problem is that, after failing at all these other "careers," the "Soccer Mom Trainer" gets the bright idea to take a 10 a.m. aerobic class at a gym. After a week or two, they get to thinking "why am I paying to do this? Why don't I have someone pay me to do this?"

And a trainer is born.

Verdict: BEWARE.

THE VOLUNTEER TURNED PROFESSIONAL

There's a bunch of nonprofit organizations out there that look for volunteers to help train people to complete a fitness event. The volunteer doesn't have to have any knowledge of fitness. Sure, if they're going to lead a group of joggers, it helps if they're a weekend runner. Going to lead a group of cyclists? Yeah, it's great if they've spent a little time on a bike. But none of these volunteers are qualified to train people. Nor do they have to be.

A while back, I was asked to ride along on one of these outings. I quickly discovered, to my horror, that there were a couple major problems with the bikes the cyclists were using. Many of the seats were wildly off, either too high or too low. In either case, that's a recipe for hip, knee and lower back problems.

But that wasn't the worst of it.

On some bikes, the skewer that clamps the wheel to the fork was dangling and loose. In other words: bad shit. Like, losing a half dozen teeth or becoming a quadriplegic bad. And you know who didn't notice that anything was wrong?

The instructor.

Truth be told, their job is to follow the script handed to them by the organization. And that's great. The problems begin when these people start thinking they actually know what they're doing and decide to spread their wings and share their wisdom among others. For money. Your money.

Once again, a trainer is born.

Verdict: BACK OUT OF THE ROOM SLOWLY

THE FRIEL EXPERT

Let's talk about Joe Friel.

This guy is the real deal. He's a qualified coach with a master's degree in exercise science. Last time I checked, this takes longer to get than an hour and a half on a computer. He's also written many books with detailed workouts to train for anything from marathons to bike racing to a triathlon. In fact, if you're a beginner aerobic athlete and you want some good advice, you can find plenty of Joe's workouts on the internet for free. He put them there. And if you want more detail, spend a couple of bucks and actually buy one of his books. You know who else did that?

This asshole.

The Friel Expert (a phrase I've coined) is a person who read Joe's books or found his free workouts on the internet, copied them, and is now selling them to you for hundreds of dollars a month. But wait, there's more! For a couple extra bucks (around a hundred of them), this jackass will actually let you speak to him for fifteen minutes a week. In fact, the whole package can often cost up to $400 dollars, depending on how much phone time you buy.

I call them the Friel Experts, but these clowns could just as easily have ripped off Hal Higdon or Chris Carmichael or any of the other legitimate fitness experts out there. Want to know something amazing? You can actually hire the real guys for about the same price.

Think about that.

You can actually hire a winning coach of Tour de France athletes for the same amount you're paying their plagiarists.

Verdict: ASSHOLES
Verdict for the real Joe Friel: THE MAN!

THE MAGAZINE TRAINER

These may be the most worthless of all the "fitness experts."

At least the Friel Expert is handing out info from Joe Friel who knows what the hell he's talking about. These nutjobs will tear a "how to get flat abs in ten minutes" article from Cosmo magazine and use it as the basis of your workout.

Here's the problem. The people writing those articles are usually not fitness experts. They're writers. You wouldn't ask a grocery bagger to perform your heart surgery, so don't ask Ernest Hemingway to come up with your ab workout.

Verdict: USELESS

THE T.A.M.

I moved to Los Angeles in 1991. Don't judge, but I spent the first couple years modeling to support myself while I worked on my training career. It turns out that this is 100 percent the opposite of what most people do. Most people try to make money in other careers, usually as waiters but sometimes as trainers, in order to support themselves while they struggle to become models and actors.

This is where we get the T.A.M.'s—the trainer/actor/model.

These people certainly look the part. Their teeth are straight and white. Their tan is perfect. Their hair is clean and shiny and they have biceps and pecs perfectly hewn from hours of gym time. But do they know how to train you?

Not only do they not know how to train you, they could care less because, in their minds, their real career as an actor/model is about to take off at any moment. Why do they think this? Because that's what some producer told them the night before as they were lured into a bedroom.

Again.

These people are only interested in themselves. Best perk of the job? The mirror in the gym so they can flex. I've often witnessed the T.A.M.s texting and taking hour-long phone calls while their clients are paying them good money.

Verdict: RUN, DON'T WALK

THE ONE-RACE EXPERT

These are people who have only done one or two races in their entire lives, which they now think makes them qualified to hang a shingle as the new expert in town. How do you spot them? Easy. They'll bring up that one race in every conversation. Example:

You: "Wow, I just had the best hamburger in L.A."

Them: "That's so funny you'd say that. When I ran the Ojai Marathon, I had the best hamburger I ever had a week later in a different town a hundred miles away."

Verdict: GO TO IN-N-OUT BURGER

THE GYM RAT

This is one of my favorite groups. These are people who love gyms. If there was a cologne called "sweat" they'd buy it. (Note to self: copyright cologne called "sweat.")

They could spend every waking hour in a gym and feel it was time well spent. And you know what? Even though many of them don't have much formal training, they usually know what the hell they're talking about. They've tried it all, done it all, and those kinds of street smarts are worth their weight in gold.

That said, keep in mind that their knowledge is varied. Their advice usually comes from trial and error on themselves. The ones with prison tattoos can probably teach you unusual techniques, like how to get a complete workout with one barbell (the big house is light on ellipticals.)

Out of all the types of trainers we've been talking about, I like these guys the best, but if you drop the soap in the shower, leave it.

Verdict: PROCEED WITH CAUTION

Now that you know how to avoid the amateur trainers, you're probably wondering how you can find the good ones. Like anything worthwhile, it's going to take some time. You have to do your homework, but there are a few guidelines.

First, a true pro trainer is most likely not going to be associated with a mega gym.

Second, a pro trainer won't advertise. If they need to advertise to get clients, you don't want them. In fact, many of the companies that hand out training certificates spend more time teaching their students how to get clients than what to do with them once they have them.

Rule of thumb: good trainers usually have a waiting list.

Third, a pro trainer won't train more than eight people a day because they'll want to spend more than an hour a day with you.

Fourth, most pro trainers have, at the very least, a degree in physical education from a major university.

Finally, anyone that claims to be a "trainer to the stars" is probably full of shit. Most pro trainers will never admit who their celebrity clients are to protect their privacy.

So where can you look for people that meet all these criteria? In a big city, try checking out the good private gyms—not the mega gyms. These boutique style gyms generally draw the better trainers, because the trainers there have to bring in their own clientele. Bottom line, if someone's driving to see this guy, you can probably assume he's pretty good.

Another place to look? Believe it or not, high schools. P.E. coaches who have lost their jobs due to cutbacks are often good trainers. Even the ones still employed might be looking for clients on the side. You can often find these guys by calling schools or asking friends with school-age kids to let you know who the good coaches are.

Finally, ask around the community to see what trainers people recommend. If the same name keeps coming up, check into the person, but make sure they've got the credentials we talked about.

That's how most people find me. Referrals from clients. And even though new clients usually meet me through my current clients, I've been surprised at how often my current clients ask me to throw a party so they can meet each other.

By the way, this could very well be the worst idea ever, and I'm including New Coke.

The last thing I need is for my worlds to collide. I wouldn't want my 10 a.m., where I end the session with the word "namaste," to mix with my 5 p.m., where we flip each other off as I leave. My clients are as different from each other as I am from that Brillo-haired, mu-mu wearing muppet Richard Simmons.

It wasn't always that way.

Thirty years ago, most of my clients were female socialites who wanted to lose weight. They didn't care about fitness routines, they didn't want to know how the sausage was made, they just wanted the weight to magically come off. Amazingly, it was often people who didn't have any weight to lose. A socialite wearing a size 2 might want to drop to a size 0.

Ten years later, I started seeing a new type of person. Businessmen who wanted to drop a suit size, mostly to impress their mistresses. The mistresses, of course, only cared about one size—and not the one you're thinking. They cared about the size of the guys' wallet.

Then, a decade later, it mutated again.

I started seeing people who wanted to get better at a particular sport: golf, tennis, running a marathon, cycling, triathlon. And they didn't want to just finish their events, they wanted to win their age group and go on to that sport's version of a National or World event. Problem was, they didn't want to spend the time to really earn it. They wanted to use their money to grease the wheels and get it the fast and easy way.

These were the same types of people that paid Sherpas in Nepal to all but piggyback them to the top of Everest so they could say "they" did it. These new kinds of clients weren't above taking steroids and other sport enhancing drugs to help them win a race. They literally would spend tens of thousands of dollars to get a medal worth three bucks.

In other words, they wanted something for nothing, which is an attitude that actually takes its biggest toll on people's health.

Chapter Thirteen
SOMETHING FOR NOTHING

IT'S EASY TO understand why we all want the quick fix, the easy way out, because we see it all around us. Talentless people get their own TV shows. Just look at the Kardashians! Quick, tell me what they're skilled at besides marrying famous athletes. They don't sing, they don't act, they don't dance, they don't do any of the things you would normally associate with talent. And yet, when Kim went through a seventy-two day marriage, it got more coverage than the tsunami in Japan.

And if adults buy into this crap, what about the most vulnerable members of our society?

Years ago, I started calling the children around me Bumper Sticker Kids. They're the kids whose parents put bumper stickers on their cars just to brag about how wonderful their children are.

"My kid is an honor student at …"

"My kid is a black-belt at …"

These are the same parents that I'd find whispering to me across the table over dinner. "My kid's special. He's in the gifted program. He takes all honor level courses. His cello teacher says he could be a prodigy."

Where are the regular dumb kids, I would wonder. The kind I grew up with? The ones like me?

It seems like every parent believes that every one of their kids is special—but if they're all special, doesn't that mean none of them are special and bring them right back to being normal?

Around this time, I noticed that many communities decided to stop keeping score during their baseball, football and soccer games because "there are no winners or losers. Everyone's a winner."

I got news for you, for someone to be a winner, someone's got to be a loser.

Unfortunately, because everyone gets participation trophies now, trophies don't mean anything any more. Spoils used to go to the victor. Now they go to everyone. Which causes two problems.

First, it teaches the loser that there's no reason to work harder to win because losing is just as good as winning.

Second, it teaches the victor "screw it, why try?" because there's no benefit to winning.

Kids aren't held accountable any more, which means they don't feel responsible for the bad things they do, which means they can't take ownership of the good things they do. And you know how this prepares them for life?

It doesn't.

These Bumper Sticker kids become adults who take no responsibility for anything. They want the quick fix, the fast cash, the easy way out. And you know what that's led to?

Thieves.

We're surrounded by predators looking to exploit this attitude of wanting something for nothing by selling you nothing for something. And you know what that something is? Your hard earned cash. And you know what the nothing they're selling is?

Diet pills. Weight loss gadgets. Supplements.

All of them are crap.

Let's talk diet pills. Or as Grace Slick would say, *Go Ask Alice.*
Ever listen to the first words in that song? Maybe you're too young.
Or, if you're old enough, maybe you were too strung out back then
to remember. Here's how it went:

> *One pill makes you larger/*
> *And one pill makes you small/*
> *And the ones that mother gives you/*
> *Don't do anything at all*

We've become a pill culture. Got a problem? Take a pill. Too
anxious during the day? Take a pill. Need to fall asleep at night? Pill
time. Want to lose weight? There's a pill for that, too—a million of
them. And what's in those pills?

Speed.

Or, at least the legal version of speed. Look on the bottle. You
probably see the words "all natural." That's the sales pitch. They
claim they're helping you lose weight the safe and "natural" way, by
speeding up your metabolism and suppressing your appetite.

So ... do they work?

Sure, for short periods, if you don't mind having the jitters
and the fact that they're terrible for your heart. You might lose a
couple pounds short term but, just like with dieting, you can't do it
long term. It's a quick fix, not a permanent fix.

Diet pills also have diminishing returns. As every drug addict
knows, your body gets used to the stuff and you need increasingly
larger doses for it to give you the same effect.

If they're so terrible, why does the FDA permit them?

Because the FDA doesn't regulate them. In fact, no one does.
Remember what FDA stands for? Food and Drug Administration.
They consider these diet pills somewhere between a food and a
drug. Neat trick, huh? Can you say "lobby"?

Historically, the only time the FDA steps in is after people die and it hits the media. As I always tell my clients:

You can't get fitness in a bottle.

Diet pills? Bad idea. But does that mean I hate everything that comes in a pill? Nope. Let me give you a quick history of vitamins.

The first one was identified in 1905. A scientist was trying to figure out why people were getting Beriberi disease on a diet of polished rice—polishing is the process they used to remove the husk. What they discovered was that the good stuff, the stuff that prevented Beriberi, was in the husk.

A couple years after that, a Polish scientist named Funk figured out that we needed certain nutrients to stay healthy. He called the nutritional parts of food "vitamine" which was later shortened to vitamin. Over the years, we've taken more and more of those good nutrients out of food, but instead of just putting them back in (which would have been too easy and sensible), we created pills to replace what was lost.

Vitamins.

Is this a bad thing? Not really, as long as you take a multi-vitamin every day. It covers you like an insurance policy, making up whatever you're missing. By the way, you don't need to get the fancy expensive brand. The grocery store brand has exactly the same stuff in it for a fraction of the cost. And, believe it or not, Flintstones has the same vitamins as the expensive one. They just add sugar.

So if you need a multi-vitamin a day, what about minerals like calcium, magnesium, chloride, sodium and potassium—otherwise known as electrolytes? Do you need more of those? Only if you're doing a job or sport that causes you to sweat a lot. Think of these as the oil in a car. You only notice it when it's gone and the engine shuts down. Same with the body. Like I tell my clients, if you're dehydrated, you're not just missing water.

So how do you replenish your electrolytes? The health food store might suggest that you need a separate bottle of each of these minerals. Please don't do that. Don't let their fake holistic kumbaya bullshit fool you into thinking they have your best interests in mind. Make no mistake, most of these health food chains are publicly traded companies that are in the business of selling you stuff. Do yourself and your wallet a favor and just get a single bottle of all-in-one capsules filled with electrolytes. Any cycling, running or sports outlets will carry them.

I'm often asked if it's possible to overdose on vitamins and electrolytes. The answer is no. It's virtually impossible if used as directed. Your body will use what it needs and the rest will become the world's most expensive pee.

But what about the rest of the stuff in the health food store?

Look at the shelves. There are literally thousands of bottles. What's in them? Do you need them? I'd like to say the answer is no but it's actually hell, no. Ever look at the guy who's trying to sell you the stuff? Does the gray hue of his skin and the sunken eyes of his vegan lifestyle look good to you?

One day I went into a health food store, and while I was picking up my multi-vitamin, the clerk asked if I needed help. Because I had some time on my hands and, well, I'm me, I decided to screw with him and said "sure." I proceeded to go up and down every aisle, pointing to bottle after bottle while asking him if I actually needed each one. The clerk's answer every time was a resounding "yes" with a detailed explanation for why I couldn't live without the pills in whatever bottle I was pointing at. When we were done, I said "So, what you're saying is, in order to live, I need one of every bottle in here?"

Finally, the guy who had an answer for everything, was stumped. He had no reply. Screw that guy.

So what kind of pills are we talking about?

Dozens of brands of plant sterols, along with hundreds of amino acids from L-Arginine to L-Tryptophan, not to mention supplemental fish oil. That's right, they squeeze the oil out of fish and want you to take it by the spoonful.

You know how else you can get fish oil? By eating fish.

Know how else you can get plant sterols? By eating plants.

Know how else you can get amino acids? By eating an egg.

All of these things we get naturally in a normal diet but, according to the clerk, in order be healthy, I needed to take one of everything in the store. They call these things supplements, but you don't need to pay absurd amounts of money to supplement anything.

You just need to eat right.

I'd like to say that health food stores have become the new drug dealers, but I can't because the products that drug dealers sell actually do something. When you buy cocaine, you can be pretty sure you're going to get high, and if you don't, you won't go back to that dealer. But when you buy L-Carnitine or fish oil capsules you don't feel any different. Are you healthier? Who the hell knows? None of these products are FDA regulated which means you're relying on the honor of a snake oil salesman.

And what's getting us to buy the most snake oil?

Infomercials!

Let's talk about a great man: Ron Popeil. Without him, we would never have had the Pocket Fisherman, Mr. Microphone and the Veg-O-Matic. Remember them? The Pocket Fisherman made fishing easy. The Veg-O-Matic made slicing and dicing vegetables a snap. And Mr. Microphone taught us how to snag chicks just like the guy in the commercial who tells the girl "Hey, good looking. I'll be back to pick you up later!"

By the way, that line doesn't work.

Ron Popeil was one-of-a-kind. When his infomercials came on, you saw the product, you knew what it did and you wanted it. Ron didn't lie. His products did make life easier.

Or at least we thought they did.

Nothing could be further from the truth when it comes to fitness products in the infomercial world. Most of them are crap and always have been. Remember the Belt Shaker? Sure, we laugh about it now, but not so long ago people thought you could actually "shake" the fat off your body.

Crazy, right?

But is that any crazier than the people today who think they can use an Electrical Stimulation Machine (E-Stim) to spot-lose fat on their stomachs? It seems crazy but there is no shortage of people out there buying products like the AbTronic that are trying to do just that.

Look, I get it. We hear about spot losing weight so much that we want to believe it's possible. Even my clients continually ask me why they can't spot lose weight. I tell them to visualize a pro cyclist. This guy is lean all over, right? But think about it, he only uses his legs to pedal. If spot losing weight were possible, only his legs would be lean.

But that's not the way it works, which doesn't stop people from trying to sell us gadgets that promise otherwise. Look at the fitness products sold on television over the past ten years. Most of them start with the word "ab". Usually ab is followed by a word like "crunch" or "energizer" or "flyer" or "rocker" or "twister"— all real products by the way. They all promise to give you washboard abs but, as I said, the only thing that can give you washboard abs is your diet.

And it's not just ab gadgets that try to sell you on spot losing weight. Think of one of the all-time top-selling pieces of fitness equipment that people hoped would do just that. If you said the

"Thighmaster" pat yourself on the back. Sure, it might build some thigh muscles, but will you spot-lose weight with it?

Forget it.

What about things like the Perfect Pushup? They say that by putting a little twist into the pushups, not only are you working your pecs and your triceps but you're also working your abs.

Really, folks?

I'm supposed to spend close to a hundred dollars on something I can do for free? Hardly any exercise in life requires less equipment than a pushup. All you need is ... the Earth. And this isn't even a crazy product.

Compare it to the Shake Weight. You've seen this ridiculous thing. The ads make it look like you get your workout by jerking off a dumbell! And yet it's selling like crazy.

But the Shake Weight looks positively effective compared to the iGallop. The concept behind this genius device? That horse-back riding is great exercise.

Absolutely true—if you're the horse.

The ad goes on to explain that not everyone has a horse, which is why you should get this horse substitute. Then we see a dozen sexy women riding this insane thing as they do a really bad impression of Debra Winger in *Urban Cowboy*. In fact, they actually wore chaps and cowboy hats in the ad while pretending to shoot finger guns.

Not to be outdone, have you seen the Range Of Motion machine, otherwise known as the "ROM" Time Machine? This device promises to give you a complete workout in just four minutes a day. Four minutes a day! That's fantastic! How much would you pay for a product that gives you a complete workout in just four minutes a day? I know I would pay a little extra for a product that did something so miraculous. So what's a good price for it? A hundred dollars? Two hundred dollars? Would you pay as much as three hundred dollars? I would!

Actual cost: around fifteen thousand dollars.

And, no, that's not a typo.

Look, the Range Of Motion machine actually does work your whole body, and it even does it in four minutes a day. The problem is that it won't get you into optimal shape in just four minutes a day. You know how I know that? Because nothing can get you there in just four minutes a day!

You'd need to spend more time with the thing ... and you'd have to have fifteen grand just lying around.

But what if you don't?

Don't worry. You're in luck. There's a product on the market right now that's actually "too good to be true!"

It works your upper body, your lower body, your core! It's a weight bearing exercise that strengthens your entire skeletal and muscular system! It's also aerobic, which is great for your cardiovascular system and helps you lose inches around the middle! And, if that's not enough, it increases both your eye/hand and eye/foot coordination!

Sold yet?

But wait, there's more!

It weighs less than a pound! It's portable and completely collapsible! Not only will it fit inside a briefcase, it will actually fit inside your shaving kit! You can take it on vacation! You can take it to the office! You can have fun with it at the beach!

Sold yet?

But wait, there's more!

It's safe and there are no moving parts to break! It's virtually indestructible! And it's so simple to use that it doesn't even need to come with instructions! It's also unisex, equally effective for both men and women! Plus, kids love it, too!

Now how much would you expect to pay for an item that does all this?

Remember, the Range Of Motion machine costs around fifteen thousand dollars, so something this spectacular should cost at least twice that, right? But it's not thirty thousand dollars. It's not even twenty thousand dollars. In fact, if you buy the very best one available, you might spend twelve.

Not twelve thousand.

Twelve dollars.

But you should really expect to pay somewhere in the neighborhood of three to five.

So what is this miraculous device? Is it a technological marvel that was recently invented by NASA for the space program? Nope. It's been around for a long time and you probably even had one when you were a kid. Want to know what it is?

A jump rope.

When my clients ask me to name the best piece of fitness equipment, I always tell them the jump rope because it does it all. It works everything and costs nothing. If you want to buy something, buy that. It delivers. Not everything does, which is why I start every podcast by saying, "Your good intentions have been stolen and I'm here to help you get 'em back."

Get ready. I feel a rant coming.

Chapter Fourteen
LET'S GET MENTAL

MAYBE YOU'VE ALWAYS been overweight.

Or maybe an extra twenty or thirty pounds have crept up on you and you want to get rid of them.

Either way, you've finally decided to do everything you can to get yourself trim, healthy and feeling great. So, with the best of intentions and a positive attitude, you buy useless supplements or crappy fitness gadgets to help you achieve your goals. They don't work and you get burned. Which isn't so terrible if it happens once or twice. But if you get burned enough times, you'll give up trying to get healthy.

Which is why these products make me so angry.

The very stuff that's supposed to be helping you is subverting your good intentions, and you're paying for the privilege! And it's not just bad food, bad drugs or bad equipment that's keeping us from being the people we want to be. Have you ever noticed how hard it is to do anything worthwhile? It's like the universe conspires to stop us from meeting our goals, from creating, from succeeding. Would you like to hear the two things that people constantly tell me they plan on doing?

Write a book.

Run a marathon.

You know how many people actually end up doing these things? Almost none. Which is crazy if you think about it. Writing a book and running a marathon cost just about exactly the same.

Nothing.

If you can afford paper, you can write a book. If you can afford shoes, you can run a marathon. Hell, you don't even really need the shoes! There's no special equipment involved. And yet, very few people who say they're going to do these things actually end up doing them. Why? There's an old saying:

> *Every morning in Africa, a gazelle wakes up. It knows it must run faster than the fastest lion or it will be killed.*
> *Every morning a lion wakes up. It knows it must outrun the slowest gazelle or it will starve to death.*
> *It doesn't matter whether you are a lion or a gazelle: when the sun comes up, you'd better be running.*
>
> —African Proverb

This is true for lions and gazelle everywhere, except one place—captivity. They don't run because they don't have to. Their food is provided for them. All they have to do is eat it. So they sit there lounging and grazing contentedly, not realizing that the price they've paid for this easy living is that they're stuck in a cage until they die.

We're the same way.

We've created a world where, for the most part, we're not going to starve, we're not going to get eaten and, as shitty as our health care system is, we're basically going to get taken care of. We don't wake up running because we don't have to.

Like the lions and gazelles in captivity, we've been trained to ignore our natural instincts to create things and move our bodies and accomplish goals, not realizing that there's a terrible price to be paid for this supposed "easy living." And the price is that we've lost the will and drive to do the big things we tell ourselves we'll get around to doing, like finish that book or run that marathon, because they don't have to be done.

But that's not the way it used to be.

Legend has it that the very first marathon was run when a Greek guy named Pheidippides was sent from the town of Marathon to Athens to announce that the Persians had been defeated. He was so excited that he ran the entire way without stopping and then collapsed from exhaustion. That's how the marathon was created. I've always thought that if they'd just given this poor bastard a horse, you'd be hard pressed to find a famous Kenyan today.

The point is, it's easy to say you're going to do something but hard to actually do it when it's not a matter of life or death, so we look for excuses not to.

In my business, I probably hear more excuses than cops and teachers combined. They get "a dog ate my homework" and "it wasn't me, officer." I get everything else. You wouldn't believe the stuff people tell me to avoid working out. I get a lot of calls from parents who say that they can't work out later that day because "I have to pick my kids up at school/soccer/friend's house."

Usually, I mess with them a little and tell them "that's no problem. I'm going to be passing by your kid's school/soccer/friend's house on the way to yours. I'll pick them up for you and then we can still work out." At this point, to get out of that, their lie just becomes bigger and more convoluted.

In fact, that reminds me of a quick story. I was heading to a client's house when she called to tell me she couldn't work out.

"Sorry, Vinnie," she said, apologetically. "But I'm stuck in traffic and I'm not going to make it home in time."

Okay, I thought. That happens. "No problem," I told her.

But she didn't stop talking, which is how I knew she wasn't Italian because, as every Italian knows, the less you talk, the better off you are.

"I'm on the 101," she continued, "and it's a parking lot right now."

Okay, I thought again. The 101 gets like that. Of course, at the time, I was on the 101 headed to her house and it didn't look like a parking lot to me, but maybe she was on a different part of it.

"Don't worry about it," I said.

But still she kept talking.

"I'm at the Reseda exit. I'm stuck here. Traffic hasn't moved an inch for ten minutes."

Funny thing was, I was on the 101 at the Reseda exit and I was doing seventy. Which reminds me of another Vinnie-ism.

If you're gonna lie, keep it simple.

I could have called her on it but that's just not something I do. Most of my clients are not lazy people. They're Hollywood types—writers, actors, directors, executives—and they often work crazy hours. Sixteen-hour days are not uncommon. So I cut them some slack, even when their excuses are long-winded and lame.

Even though they don't need to write an opera to explain why they don't want to work out, there's one excuse that's a guaranteed "Get Out Of Workout Free" card with me. If they say they have a physical ailment of any sort—back pain, a pulled muscle, a severe headache—I have to respect it. I may be a lie detector, but I'm not an MRI machine.

If someone complains of a physical problem, as far as I'm concerned, as a professional, it's game over. They can work out another day. Their health is my number one priority.

Which brings up another point.

Because so many of my clients are creative types, I see a lot of drug use. It's no secret that Hollywood and drugs go hand in hand. It's not my moral obligation to judge my client's pharmaceutical escapades, but I always demand to know what they're on. If I hear any sort of speed, coke or meth, the workout's off and it means we're going to spend the next hour hanging out and talking. If they took a downer, I'll usually help them get undressed and put them to bed, even if it's noon.

But crazy and convoluted excuses aren't the only ones I get. I also hear a lot of simple, stupid ones. You wouldn't believe how many times I've heard these to avoid working out:

"I have a hangnail."

"I have to wash my hair."

And (my favorite) *cough, cough*, "I think I'm getting sick."

The *cough, cough* always makes me laugh. But the excuse I probably hear most often, in a hundred different flavors, is that people just don't have "the time"—which is odd because we have more time saving devices in our lives now than at any other point in the history of the world. We don't have to catch, kill, butcher or grow our own food any more. Let's face it, hunting, fishing and gardening is what we do now to relax.

But I get it.

We lead busy lives and it's difficult to find the time to keep up a workout schedule. And time is not the only obstacle we face. What about negativity? We're constantly bombarded with it. Once you start losing weight and getting fit, what do the people around you say?

Sure, some will be positive.

"You look great!"

But others won't be so kind.

"You're getting too thin! You look unhealthy!"

"Be careful about putting on all that muscle. It's going to turn to fat!"

I helped my nephew drop over sixty pounds in just under five months and he looked and felt better than he ever had in his life. But what did the people around him say?

"You're too thin! You need to put some of that weight back on!"

Bear in mind, at this point he was still a good ten pounds above his optimal weight. People were quick to tell him that he wasn't eating healthy and he should go back to eating like they do.

"Who are these people?" I asked.

"My friends. Co-workers and family," he replied. Then he realized something. "You know what? Everyone who tells me that stuff is obese."

He told me that his new way of eating wasn't difficult to follow, the hard part was the people around him making it difficult. They would literally try to sabotage him by taking him to pizza joints to get him to eat food he knew was going to be bad for him. He asked me why they were doing this.

"You're basically holding up a mirror to everyone around you," I told him. "And they don't like what they see. Because you're succeeding, they see themselves as failures."

He wanted to know what he should say to everyone so he could help educate them. I told him to say nothing. Just do your thing. Lead by example. Or, to give you another Vinnie-ism (God help me):

Nobody wants to hear it. Everyone wants to see it.

He ended up leading by example and is now looking and feeling great.

Don't let all the negativity make you lose your enthusiasm— or, as Robert DeNiro pronounces it in the baseball bat scene in *The Untouchables* (one of the greatest scenes in movie history) "En-two-siasm!" Know this: there will always be speed bumps on your road to fitness, and they will never go away, no matter how in shape you get. You will always find things you have to overcome. In fact, you'll find that those obstacles will appear even more frequently as you continue on your path, and that they'll crop up in the places you least expect.

Friends and family. The workplace. The old injury that rears its ugly head.

There will always be something that will try to unhinge your forward progress, and that brings us to a larger point.

Fitness is more a mental game than a physical one.

When I try to motivate my clients, they often tell me that I don't understand what they're going through, that working out is difficult for them but easy for me because I've been doing it my whole life. The underlying point, I guess, is that I'm somehow immune to the kind of obstacles they face.

I'm not.

It's not something I particularly love to talk about, but I haven't held anything back from you yet and I'm not going to start now. Trust me, I have real skin in the game—a game that, for me, was literally life or death. Up till now, I've kept this stuff relatively private, but God hates a coward, right?

Settle in and let me tell you about it.

Part Three

LIFE INTO LIVING

Chapter Fifteen
SKIN IN THE GAME

A HOT GIRL named Jayne got me into cycling.

I was twenty-one years old and we were on a date at the Camellia Grill in uptown New Orleans. Over one of their spectacular chili-cheese omelets, I mentioned that the dryer at the laundromat must be broken because my jeans were shrinking. She smirked and told me that my jeans were fine, I was just getting fat. I, of course, knew that was impossible, because I'd always told myself that I'd never be one of those ex-football players who grew a gut. But the truth was in the numbers. After I finished playing college football, I was a ripped two hundred and forty pounds. Somehow that slim two-forty crept up to a jolly two-seventy in no time.

Jayne was right. I was getting fat.

That night, I checked myself out in the mirror and, sure enough, I saw a gut, plain as day. How had I missed it? I decided I needed to do something about it, so I went straight to Jayne for help. She was a pro at this. Jewish girls from Long Island basically invented dieting. Case in point, the woman who started Weight

Watchers was a housewife from that area. Jayne was an expert on losing weight. I asked her how to do it.

"Well, there's the Dexetrim and Tab diet," she told me. "Or you could try the coke diet."

"You just drink diet coke?" I asked.

"No, you diet by snorting coke."

I decided to go with the Dexetrim and Tab diet. Seemed cheaper. So I went to the drug store and bought some of each. On my way home, I popped two pills (the box said to just take one but I'm a big guy) and I chased it down with a Tab. By the time I got home, I was a jittery, shaky mess. I called Jayne and told her I was about to crawl out of my skin.

"You're only supposed to take one," she said. "But don't worry, you'll get used to the jitters after a while."

It turned out, that was the way I was supposed to feel on that diet. I decided I couldn't live like that, so I went back to the store and bought every magazine that promised to tell how to lose ten pounds in ten minutes.

By the way, let me tell you something about them. Those articles are complete crap. In fact, if you look at a year's worth of articles in the same fitness magazine, you'll see how they contradict each other.

Here's an example. Running magazines used to preach that you should buy thick-soled running shoes with lots and lots of cushion and stabilizers … until barefoot running came into fashion. Unfortunately, magazines survive on advertising and they can't sell you bare feet. So the shoe companies started making "minimalist" shoes that they claimed were better than bare feet, which is kind of like beverage companies telling you that their drink quenches your thirst better than water. After that, those same magazines started writing articles preaching about how you should now buy lightweight running shoes.

Anyway, pretty soon it became clear that the magazine's "professional" advice was bullshit. In fact, I was shocked to discover that they were just out and out lying. So with the Dexetrim and Tab diet shot and the magazines not working, I went back to my medical textbooks from college. Turned out that they had a really radical approach.

Eat sensibly and exercise.

Who would have thunk it?

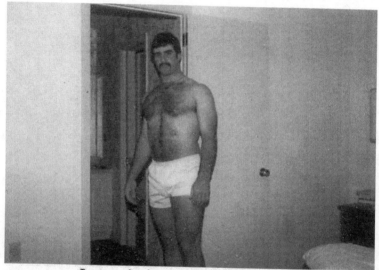

Twenty pounds under my heaviest weight and the first time I felt comfortable taking my shirt off in front of people.

At the time, I was careful with how I spent my money—mostly because I hardly had any. Like most Italians, I had a pizza budget. So I decided to kill two birds with one stone by taking my pizza money and using it to buy a bike, a maroon Fuji. From that point on, if I had to go anywhere, I rode there on the bike. In fact, to this day, when people tell me they don't have time to exercise, I tell them to make their manner of conveyance their exercise.

They're usually surprised I know a word like "conveyance" and sometimes they even listen to me.

So that's what got me into biking.

I wasn't doing it as a sport yet, it was purely a way to lose weight. And it worked—but not exactly in the way I thought. Sure, the exercise from the bike helped me to drop pounds but, more importantly, the money I spent on the bike no longer went toward buying pizza, junk food and the rest of the sugary crap I'd been surviving on. Not only had I added aerobic exercise, I'd improved my diet.

My goal was to drop down to my usual weight of two-forty. After three months, I was surprised to find that I'd dropped even further. The scale said two-thirty. And it happened without me even noticing. I wasn't consciously exercising or dieting. I was just riding around, living my life, eating properly for the first time and, next thing I knew, I was down to two-ten. Hell, I didn't even realize I was at that weight until my clothes stopped fitting and I had to get my jeans taken in.

Even though losing weight was my initial goal, I ended up being a lot more interested in the bike, which I'd always previously thought of as a child's toy. Riding around on it was oddly liberating. New Orleans had always been a tourist city and its streets were jammed with streetcars and tour buses. If I wanted to drive my car all the way from uptown, down to Cafe Du Monde in the French Quarter during the middle of the day, it would take an hour. But, on my bicycle, weaving in and out of traffic, I could whiz down, have a coffee and be back uptown in the same hour.

The only time I didn't ride my bike was when I went to visit my parents in Donaldsonville—an eighty mile one-way trip through the swamp. For that, I always used to take my car. But one day, I decided to give it a shot on my bike. What the hell, right? How long could it take? The answer: three and a half hours. Unless you get dragged off the bike by a gator. Or pelted with beer cans by rednecks in a truck.

I'm not kidding.

Back then, hardly anyone had seen the tight European bike shorts that everyone wears now. And you know what area had really not seen them? The swamps of Louisiana. So when I rode to my parents wearing my lycra bike shorts, it was not uncommon for good old boys in their pick-up trucks to hurl bottles at me and call me a faggot. And you know what I was thinking when they were doing that?

Whew! At least they didn't shoot me!

That, by the way, was when I started wearing a helmet. Helped defend against the beer bottles. You think I'm kidding.

So that's how biking would have stayed for me—an enjoyable hobby and a great way to get around until, somewhere around the mid-eighties, I read about a guy named Pete Penseyres. He'd just done one of the most miraculous athletic feats on a bike that I'd ever heard about. Pete completed the RAAM (the Race Across America) in eight days, nine hours and forty-seven minutes with an average speed of 15.4 mph. That probably means nothing to you, but here's how amazing it is: as I write this, that record still holds.

I became obsessed with RAAM. I had to know more about it. Who could do it? How did you sign up for it? Of course, in 1986 there was no Google, so information was almost impossible to come by—unless you wanted to go to a library, but those places are rarely dripping with hot chicks, so I stayed away. Instead, I grabbed every article I could find, sometimes ordering out-of-date magazines, even if they only had a word or two about Penseyre's incredible feat.

Even more amazing than the actual time he spent crossing the continent was the amount of time he slept each day.

Less than ninety minutes every twenty-four hours. The rest of the time he was on that bike. It was his life. Back then, the longest I'd ever ridden in a single stretch was the eighty miles to my parent's house. And when I finished that ride, I was always tired. So tired, in fact, that I'd sleep over at their place so that I didn't have to tackle the return trip until after I'd gotten a full night's rest.

During the RAAM, Pete Penseyres biked for over twenty-four hours straight. And he wasn't even the only one doing it. Who are these guys, I thought? How is such a thing even humanly possible?

If they could do it, why not me?

It seemed like the only way to even have a shot at getting into that kind of shape was to take a year off and train night and day. Unfortunately, I wasn't born with the last name Trump and P.E. teachers (which is how I earned my living at the time) don't make anywhere near enough to just casually take a year off to train for something like that.

But I had to do something.

At the time, for extra money, I hosted a local radio show as well as had a stable of clients that I got paid to train. I was the only game in town. Life was good.

But it wasn't great.

It rained a lot in Louisiana. And it was hot and humid. And there were no mountains to speak of—something that seemed critical if I was going to train really hard. But I knew of a place that didn't have any of those problems. And I figured there was enough wealth there that I could pick up enough new clients to survive.

Los Angeles.

So I got in my Toyota Forerunner and started driving. Anything that didn't fit, I left behind. I told myself I wasn't going to stop until I arrived. I figured if Pete Penseyres could bike for twenty-four hours straight, I could certainly drive for that long. Also, I was afraid that if I stopped anywhere and spent the night, I would wake up remembering my cozy little life back in Louisiana, wonder what the hell I was doing, then turn around and drive home.

So I went straight through. The trip took thirty-five hours.

As I settled into my new life in Southern California, I began looking for super long distance ultra events to compete in. I started with a twelve-hour mountain bike race. Believe it or not, it was tough to find one that long. At the time, most races lasted only ninety minutes. The conventional wisdom was that significantly longer ones were too dangerous.

Didn't matter. I was desperate to ride in it.

The problem was that it was only two months away—not a lot of time to get ready. But I knew if I missed this one, I'd have to wait a whole year before it was held again, which meant I had to figure out a way to ramp up my training regimen quickly. So I joined Bally's and 24-Hour Fitness figuring that, no matter where I was, I could at least find a gym nearby stocked with lifecycles. Whenever I wasn't with a client, I rode, even if it was only for an hour or two. Weekends were a different story. I pedaled my bike into the Santa Monica mountains for as long as I could manage. I worked up to twelve or thirteen hours at a stretch.

Finally, I was ready. Or at least I thought I was.

The race took place in Big Bear, CA in the San Bernadino mountains. As I drove to the event the day before the race, I realized that I had made a critical error. Big Bear's elevation was over six thousand feet, but the race climbed into the mountains much higher. Even though I always acclimated well to altitude, I couldn't do it overnight. I wasn't prepared.

The race started at 7 a.m. on a cold, crisp August morning. I'd hoped that the heat would hold off until mid-afternoon, but it ended up getting dog hot by 9 a.m. Even though there were around one hundred people making the climb, most of them were in the tag-team competition. Only about twenty of us mutants were insane enough for the solo competition, trying to see how many laps up and down the mountain we could complete in twelve straight hours.

The uphills were steep and grueling but the downhills were even worse—a single track down loose shale rock. I got one good piece of advice before the race from a guy named Will. He and his brother, Owen, own Universal Cycles in L.A., my local bike shop. "Don't use the brakes on the downhill," he told me. "They are not your friend."

He was mostly right. You can use the back brakes a little and you'll only end up slipping and sliding—I learned that in the Santa Monica mountains, also known as the bunny slopes. Problem is, the back brakes don't do much in the way of actually stopping you. Only the front brake can do that. Unfortunately, if you actually use the front brake, you'll go head over handlebars quicker than you can think.

I learned that little trick on my first lap of the race.

Luckily, I had a good fall, meaning I was able to get back up and my bike was okay. Since we're on the subject, would you like to know the secret to stopping on a steep downhill? Okay, here it is—don't.

The race was brutal. It would have been tough for an experienced mountain biker on a pro bike, but I was a roadie on a borrowed bike who hadn't given himself enough time to acclimate to the altitude and who didn't have enough sense to avoid killing himself.

Around the seven-hour mark, I was exhausted, depleted and feeling flu-like symptoms. But, to me, this seemed like good news. Surely, this was how Pete Penseyres felt when he set his remarkable record, right? To be a true champion, you had to just push through the pain. Or so I thought.

I forced myself onward, not realizing that the reason I was exhausted was because I was only eating a single power bar every hour. It wasn't nearly enough to fuel me. And the reason I was feeling flu-like was because I had completely sweated out my electrolytes without replenishing them. In short, I was starving and dehydrated.

Later, I would learn that the prevailing wisdom was that you needed to take in anywhere from two hundred and fifty to three hundred calories an hour to keep yourself fueled. That was based on the calorie in/calorie out concept, which demanded that you replenish the calories you were burning so you could keep going.

And how did they want you to get those calories?

Largely through nutrition bars, gels and sports drinks. In other words, through sugar and grains.

Had I known then what I know now, I would have thrown that whole bullshit concept out the window and done what you're supposed to do, which is eat a high fat diet while staying away from sugars and grains, allowing my body to get its fuel from it's preferred source. Fat.

Unfortunately, at the time, there was no study or doctor anywhere telling you to eat that way during an endurance event. They wanted you to get your calories from sugar, which is bad enough. And, to make matters worse, during this race, I wasn't even doing that!

I was starving.

My body was shutting down.

Even worse than the lack of nutrition was the fact that I was incredibly dehydrated. You need to drink anywhere from sixteen to twenty-four ounces of water, along with electrolytes, depending on how hot it is outside.

I wasn't drinking anywhere near enough.

But I pushed on, biking like hell. I gave it everything I had, humping the bike like a monkey trying to fuck a football. Time crept agonizingly by. I felt like a school kid watching the seconds slowly tick away, waiting for the three o'clock bell.

By the tenth hour, I was in so much pain I couldn't even figure out where it was coming from any more. Everything hurt. Even

my hair and fingernails hurt and they don't even have nerve endings. To make matters worse, in this type of race, you never knew
your position in the pack, so I just assumed I was way behind,
which spurred me to try even harder. The only thing that got me
through the last couple hours was a Chuck Berry song called *Never
Can Tell*. One line kept running through my head in an endless
loop.

> *"C'est la vie" say the old folks,*
> *it goes to show you never can tell …*

Eventually, thankfully, it was over.

I got off my bike at the finish line to see two guys laying on
their backs on the asphalt. I wondered what was wrong with them,
then I took a step and found out. I collapsed, unable to stand or
even move.

I had come in third.

True, those guys had beaten me but it turned out they were
sponsored pros. They did this all the time.

Later, I would discover that I had driven them crazy because
they knew I was always right behind them, forcing them to go
harder than they usually rode. Laying there on the hot asphalt, I
realized two things.

First, this was the most pain I had ever felt in my entire life.

And second, I couldn't wait to get back on the bike and find
another race.

Chapter Sixteen
THE TOUGHEST FORTY-EIGHT HOURS IN SPORTS

ONCE THE ULTRA bug bites you, it doesn't go away.

I quickly moved from twelve-hour races to twenty-four hour races and I really stepped up my training program. I bought a Schwinn Spinner. There wasn't enough room for it in my apartment, so I got rid of my couch. I rode it every hour I was home. If I was by a gym, I'd go in and ride their Lifecycles. On weekends, I'd hit the Santa Monica mountains and ride until I couldn't go any more.

There was a surprising side benefit to this obsession. Clients who often complained that there weren't enough hours in the day to fit in their workouts, saw what I was doing and stopped complaining. I led by example. Some of them were even in shape enough to ride with me for a couple hours.

I was an animal. Within a couple years, twenty-four hour mountain bike racing became a big deal, with spectators and sponsors, and I was on the circuit doing my thing. Eventually, in the late nineties, a company called 24 Hours of Adrenaline hosted the first world twenty-four hour mountain bike race and I was invited along with forty other athletes from around the world. Also competing was Wolfgang Fasching, that year's RAAM winner.

I beat him … sort of.

He quit after fourteen hours. I don't know why. It just goes to show that there's no guarantees. Two hours later, I crashed out myself after having blacked out on the bike. This was becoming a common problem for me. The shoulder injury I'd gotten playing college football had steadily worsened over the years and the bouncing of the mountain bike filled it with such agony that I sometimes blacked out while training. I fell off the bike and ended up with a concussion, but at least I'd beaten the RAAM winner. I guess that's my way of putting a shine on a turd.

But then I faced a real dilemma. Blacking out while riding is a dangerous problem and doing it while flying thirty-five miles per hour down steep, rocky terrain is a death sentence. Reluctantly, I gave up the mountain bike.

And focused on my road bike.

It required just as much endurance but with less pounding, which spared my shoulder and kept me conscious. And I kept training. I rode all the time. To the coffee shop and back. Forty mile rides. Hundred mile rides. Didn't matter. I couldn't stop. I was obsessed with the idea of going long. Soon, I found myself biking until sunup, looking for races that were more and more extreme.

And if there weren't any races available, I'd make up my own challenges.

I wanted to do a three hundred mile race but I couldn't find one, so I rode my bike from Los Angeles to Santa Barbara and back, taking a long mountain route that ended up just over three hundred miles. If I wasn't with clients, I was on the bike or the spinner, building my aerobic base. I was so busy, I didn't date as much as I used to. I was in love with going long.

My friends saw this and were getting concerned. When I'd tell them how long these races were or how hard I'd been training, they'd think that I was either lying or needed help. In fact, it got to the point that I did lie about the length of my rides. I'd pretend I was doing less distance than I really was. Whenever anyone asked me how far I rode, my standard answer was seventy miles. That always seemed long enough to be plausible but not so long that they'd think I was crazy.

But that didn't work on one of my friends. She was so convinced that I had some kind of mental disorder that she insisted I go see her three-hundred-dollar-an-hour psychiatrist on her dime. I went, only to prove that I wasn't crazy.

The session lasted three hours. Nine hundred dollars later, the psychiatrist had a diagnosis. He said that, in most things, I was perfectly normal but that he thought I had Obsessive Compulsive Disorder, along with Social Anxiety Disorder. Turns out there's medication for that stuff, which he said he could prescribe. I asked him what the medicine would do.

"You know how you go on a bike ride for ten hours?" he said. "Well, on this medicine, after five hours, you might feel like you've gone far enough and stop and go enjoy something else and you'd feel fine about it."

I stared at him. If you've never seen me stare, it's unnerving. "Let me ask you something," I said. "How long have these drugs been around?"

"Oh, twenty or thirty years or so."

I nodded. "It's a good thing they weren't around a couple hundred years ago or DaVinci might have blown off finishing the Mona Lisa so he could go enjoy a gelato instead."

The psychiatrist thought about that. "You might be right."

So what if I'm a little crazy? I'd argue that anyone who ever did anything worth doing is probably a little crazy. In any event, I never took the drugs, which was a good thing because they probably would have prevented me from tackling my new obsession.

The Furnace Creek 508.

Even then it was legendary, the toughest race west of the Mississippi. Hell, one of the toughest in the world. It was billed as "the toughest 48 hours in sports" and it was designed by a psychopath. His name is Chris Kostman. I sometimes find myself imagining how he must have described it to the first participant.

"Okay, I have this idea for a race. You're gonna love it. It's going to last over five hundred miles. Nonstop. No sleep. No rest. But you have to complete the whole thing in forty-eight hours or you're disqualified.

"I see you shaking your head but, wait, it gets better.

"During the race, you're going to have to climb a vertical mile to the top of a mountain before descending at dizzying speed to the lowest point in the Western Hemisphere. You guessed it, Death Valley. It's called that because the conditions there are so horrible that hardly anything but snakes and scorpions can survive.

"The good news is, you won't be doing that in the heat of the day.

"The bad news is, you'll arrive in the middle of the night, when it's pitch black.

"You'll pass by a fart of a town called Furnace Creek and, because the race is called The Furnace Creek 508, you'll be tempted to think that's the finish line. But that's just me screwing with you. That's just the mid-way point.

"Ha ha.

"So you'll ride all night long through Death Valley and, when the sun comes up, you'll be shocked to discover you're still in Death Valley. That should really screw with you.

"And that climb over the mountain to get into Death Valley in the first place? That's not the only climb in the race. In fact, you'll cumulatively climb over thirty-five thousand feet. Would you like to know how high Mt. Everest is?

"Twenty-nine thousand feet.

"That's right. During this race, you will bike higher than Everest. And you'll do it in scorching heat, with sixty-mile-an-hour winds and, in some cases, flash floods. And the kicker is, if you make it to the end, when the finish line is in sight, you won't be able to coast to it because I'm going to stick it half-way up a damn hill!

"But that's not even the final insult.

"Even though I'm calling the race The 508, it's really 509 and a half miles. You need to go that extra mile and a half just so I can end it on a hill. And, when you finish—if you do, but you probably won't—there won't be any cash prize waiting for you, there won't be any fanfare, we won't even spring for proper "finish-line" tape for you to break through. We'll just steal some toilet paper from the shitty hotel. Ha ha!

"So ... what do you think?"

Well, this is what I thought: "Where do I sign up?"

But, before I did, I wanted to experience it. So I went on the internet to see if any of the upcoming racers needed someone to crew for them. I found three people. Two women and this guy named David Holt.

Now, don't get angry, but my thinking at the time was that the women would probably end up crying and I had no idea how to deal with crying women, so I picked the guy. I met him for the first time the day before the race.

I was expecting a rock hard Adonis, a muscular athlete capable of tackling one of the toughest courses on Earth.

What I found was a hunched guy with bad posture who looked like Woody Allen and Abe Vigoda had a kid. He was in his mid-fifties, gentle and soft-spoken. How is this guy ever going to finish this race, I thought? What I didn't realize was that the previous year, he not only finished the race, he came in second. And not just second in his age group—second in the whole damn thing.

David Holt, it turned out, was a badass.

Watching him during the race was an education. Not only did I learn the course, I learned all the other things that you can only discover by having a front row seat—how to choose a crew, how to organize the van, where the winds picked up, how to handle the searing heat and freezing cold. Even though David didn't look like an athlete, he was one. He had heart. He was steady. Hour after hour, on one of the most treacherous courses around, he kept going like an Energizer bunny with oversized batteries. He never stopped. He never quit.

When it was over, he ended up finishing eighth in a field that included pro and Olympic athletes. It was inspiring and we formed a great friendship. I'd hoped to train with him as I got ready to compete in The Furnace Creek 508 the following year, which would take place in October. He was happy to oblige and we got together whenever we could.

I started training. Hard.

Beginning in January, I pedaled my bike to my client's houses to make sure I spent as much time in the saddle as possible. That month, I spent fifty hours on the bike. In February, sixty. Every month I kept adding hours and distance until, by the end of April, I'd logged over five thousand miles.

By July and August, I was racking up nearly two thousand miles a month, including twenty-four hour periods where I rode without stopping for sleep or rest.

Finally, in October, I was ready.

I wasn't looking for a win. I wasn't even looking to keep up with the veterans, like David Holt. My goal was to simply have a strong finish, hopefully somewhere in the top ten.

The race started just after dawn at the Hilton Garden Inn in Santa Clarita, on a cool, clear October morning.

It ended in Death Valley the following morning as the sun began to peek over the horizon. I had DNFd—an ultra term for "Did Not

Finish" or, jokingly, "Did Nothing Fatal." I had made it almost three quarters of the way through the course when my knee gave out.

It first started bothering me in Trona, a little town notable only for the taco stand that stood about a hundred and seventy miles into the race. I felt a dull soreness in my left knee. I'd never experienced that before. I'd only been on the bike for about eight hours, so I pushed through it.

For the next several hours, it came and went and I thought I could handle it, but it really started to get my attention in Townes Pass, which is the thirteen-mile climb over the mountain range that drops into Death Valley on the other side. The grade there was between 10 and 13 percent. If you're not sure how steep that is, get on a treadmill and set the incline to thirteen.

Now you see what I'm talking about.

As I gutted my way up the mountain, the dull pain became a roar, which culminated in a popping sensation that felt like a tendon had pulled away from the bone. I kept going, descending into Death Valley as the sun went down, flying at fifty-miles-an-hour into a dark abyss.

When I finally got to the mid-way point at Furnace Creek, I wrapped my knee in ice, took a handful of Advil and continued on, pedaling all night and into the morning. By then, I was in such agony that I couldn't even lift my knee high enough to get my foot to the top of the pedal stroke. I began to wonder if I was doing permanent damage to the joint.

As the sun came up, I had a "come to Jesus" meeting with Mehran, my crew chief. The rules stipulated that, as long as you and the bike stayed together, you could get off and push it to the finish line. Mehran calculated how long it would take me to finish if I pushed the bike up the hills and cruised down the back sides. The math was clear. It would take about a month. There was no way I could do that and finish before the forty-eight hour time limit, which would disqualify me.

Between that, and the concern over the permanent damage I was in danger of doing to my knee, I made one of the hardest choices of my life. I've never been a quitter. It's not in my DNA. Even so, the facts were the facts. I had to be smart about it. Also not in my DNA.

I dropped out of the race.

This was a race I'd spent a year to train for and a lifetime to prepare for. I was devastated. Even worse, I felt like I'd let my crew down. Adam Zelinsky and Mehran Salamati had given up their entire weekend, not to mention a night's sleep, just to see me cross the finish line.

But then, another thought crept into my mind, a simpler and truer one—screw it. It's just a race. In the grand scheme of things, it didn't really mean anything. How could I be so narcissistic as to care about something as stupid as crossing a finish line when I knew there were kids, right then, with life-threatening illnesses lying in bed in St. Jude Children's Hospital—some of whom wouldn't live to see another sunrise?

It put everything in perspective.

So I dropped out. But I didn't quit. The next year I signed up again and trained relentlessly for seven months to get ready. I was convinced that this time I was going to beat this thing.

By the summer of 2007, I was in the best shape of my life. My resting heart rate was in the mid-thirties—the average for a man my age was in the seventies. My body fat percentage was below 3 percent. One doctor joked that I was so lean he could almost see the mitochondria swimming beneath my skin.

I was in phenomenal athletic shape. I was ready.

I tell you all that not to brag, but so you'll understand what a shock it was to find out I was nearly dead.

Chapter Seventeen
SOMETIMES YOU GET THE BEAR, SOMETIMES THE BEAR GETS YOU

I FOUND OUT I was dying like this.

There was a training regimen going around at the time among top pro athletes called the "sleep high, train low" method. The idea was that you would sleep at high altitudes but train at low altitudes because spending time at high altitudes increases your red blood cell count. This is good because red blood cells carry oxygen to your muscles, which increases your energy and stamina. When you hear about blood doping in cycling or the Olympics, this is what they're trying to accomplish.

But doping is illegal, not to mention bad for your health.

This wasn't.

There's a device called a hypoxic altitude tent that's basically a clear, square tent you put around your bed that makes your body react as if you were at altitude. I wanted to try using it to see if it would give me a competitive edge for the Furnace Creek 508 but, as you might imagine, they're not cheap.

Luckily, I had a plan.

I'd convinced one of the companies that make the tents to give me one if I endorsed their product, but I was only going to do that if I was certain it worked. The plan was to check my red blood cell count before I started sleeping in the tent and then, three months later, check it again to see if there was a change. If I saw a significant rise in levels, I'd know it was effective.

So I went to my friend, who's also a top Beverly Hills doctor, to get my first baseline test done. Let's call her Deborah, not because it's her real name, but because I've always liked that name. Even though I'm pretty much an open book, I figure my friend might like a little privacy.

A few days after I gave the blood sample for the baseline, I got a call from Deborah. "Honey," she said, "I got your test results back."

"Yeah, great. Just leave them at the front desk and I'll come by and pick them up."

"No, no. You have a problem. Your blood is all whacked out. Your red and white cell counts are very low."

This didn't alarm me. I thought I knew what the problem was. "You know, Deborah, I came in and gave blood after a four hour bike ride in the heat. My blood was probably just dehydrated."

"Dehydration usually makes the critical numbers go up," she said. "That means your numbers are probably even lower than they look on these results. We need to get more tests."

"Okay, I'll come in and your people can draw more blood."

"No," she said. "I'm sending you to a doctor who specializes in this."

Even though I didn't say it, there was no way in hell I was going to another doctor. So my blood was whacked? So what? Nobody's perfect. I've never really been a doctor guy. I know you're supposed to get routine checkups, but the only routine I have with checkups is not to get them. Unfortunately, Deborah knew me well enough to know that's what I was thinking, so she made the appointment herself, figuring I wouldn't disappoint someone who went out of their way for me.

And that's how I found myself in the offices of a famous TV doctor. Trust me, you've seen him. Aside from being on TV, he's worked with a lot of professional and Olympic athletes. You don't even have to ask him about it. He'll tell you.

It usually takes a long time to get any kind of doctor appointment in Beverly Hills, but because Deborah is one of the top radio oncologists in the city, I found myself in the TV doc's office the next day, getting the star treatment. They took, no exaggeration, somewhere between twenty-five and thirty vials of blood, along with every other sample he could think of. They also did a complete body scan using some sort of multi-bazillion dollar machine, which spits out statistics like your muscle density, bone density and body fat to an absurdly exacting percentage.

Finally, the TV doc entered.

He walked in with a swagger, too cool for the room, then shook my hand and said "I couldn't wait to come meet the guy with a lower body fat percentage than me." Even though he had yet to send the gallons of blood he took from me to a lab, he already had a theory as to what was wrong.

People who train as intensely as I do—between twenty-five and thirty hours a week—sometimes excrete blood through their small intestine, which comes out in their fecal matter. His theory, I guess, was that the blood I was losing through my small intestine explained my low blood cell count. Or something. I couldn't completely follow the logic.

In any event, he wanted even more samples.

That night, I was having dinner at Deborah's house. She wanted to know how things went with the TV doc and I told her that he had a theory that required extensive investigation into possible abnormalities in my fecal matter. Actually, what I really said was, "He wants to play with my poopy." She wanted to know why and I told her his theory. Before I could even finish explaining, she threw down her fork in disgust. I thought she was angry because we were talking about excrement during dinner, but it turned out she was upset for an entirely different reason.

"He totally missed it," she said, burying her face in her hands.

"Missed what?" I asked. "If you already know what's wrong with me, why am I fucking around with TV doctors?"

"I'm a radio oncologist," she said. "Blood is not my expertise. But I know enough to know you have a real problem and he's not going to find it in your toilet. That's it, you're going to see Anne."

"Anne? Who's this genius? What TV show is she on?"

Deborah rolled her eyes. "She's not on any TV show, although there is one that exactly describes doctors like her."

Yeah. You guessed it. *House.*

Next day, I'm in Dr. Anne's office—not her real name, by the way. As I sat in her waiting room, I was surprised to discover that I was surrounded by very sick people. They looked gaunt and frail. Some had yellowing skin.

What the hell am I doing here, I thought? I'm not like these people. I just rode six hours on the bike this morning! I'm in great shape!

Next thing I knew, they brought me in to see Dr. Anne.

I was expecting to find someone like Deborah, a type-A Beverly Hills go-getter. Instead, I was surprised to meet Deborah's polar opposite. Anne was soft-spoken, slightly distracted. She always seemed to be doing two or three things at once, which was understandable considering how busy her waiting room was. She reminded me of the girl next door, if the girl next door was board certified in medical oncology and internal medicine.

Dr. Anne had a gentleness about her. I instantly fell in love.

"So how do you know Deborah?" she asked.

Everybody kept asking me that question, which struck me as odd because I'd been close friends with Deborah for over twelve years and no one in her circle seemed to know who the hell I was. But I guess it made sense. Along with being a friend of mine, Deborah was also a client and I rarely socialize in public with my clients, mostly because everyone always wants to ask me about the celebrities I train. As a rule, I never talk about them to preserve their privacy, so it's easier to just avoid the social scene altogether.

So Anne took a small amount of blood and sent it off to have some preliminary tests done right away. While I was waiting for the results, Deborah walked in. That's odd, I thought, knowing how busy her schedule is. For Deborah to show up in person meant that she thought something was really wrong.

For the first time, I felt a sinking feeling.

Soon enough, the three of us were given copies of my initial test results. To me, it was like reading hieroglyphics. Out of nervousness, I started asking questions.

"Give it to me straight. Do I have hep?"

Anne, squinting at my results, said, "we can't rule it out."

"What about AIDS? I have AIDS?"

She looked up at me. "Are you homosexual or an intravenous drug user?"

I shook my head. "No."

"Lots of partners?"

I paused, but she clearly wanted an answer. "Well … yeah."

"Then we can't rule it out."

That response was starting to piss me off. "If I said 'common cold,' would you say, 'we can't rule it out'?"

But before Anne could answer, Deborah piped up. "Anne, you know what we have to do here."

Anne nodded. "Yes, but we might as well stick to procedure. Wait until all of the blood tests come back."

"But you know the blood test is going to tell us to do it anyway, so let's just do it."

"What are we talking about here?" I asked, growing frustrated. "Do what?"

Anne turned to me. "A bone marrow biopsy."

"Okay," I said with a shrug, although I wasn't really thinking about what that meant. "Let's do it."

Anne began to hem and haw. "Actually, I have them done at Cedars. I don't do them here any more. Besides, my nursing staff is already gone for the day."

"I'll assist," Deborah said, insistent.

Anne shook her head. "It's late. I have an appointment I have to get to and it would take too long to give him the sedative."

Here's something you should know about me. I've always had a high pain tolerance. When I was playing high school football and broke my leg so badly that the doctor described it as powder because it was shattered in so many places, I never had a single painkiller for it. And all of my shoulder surgeries? Same thing. Not one painkiller. You want to talk dental work? I've had my share of fillings and caps over the years. Not one shot.

I told you that to tell you this.

Because of my natural resistance to pain, when Anne said they didn't have time to give me a sedative, I shrugged and said, "Let's just do it cold."

This turned out to be a case where my alligator mouth got my bird brain into trouble. When they said sedative, in my mind I was thinking Vicodin or Percocet. You know, the kind of stuff Elvis put in his peanut butter and banana sandwiches. I later realized that when they said sedative, they were talking more like the Michael Jackson kind—the stuff that knocks you out. If I'd thought about it even a second more, I would have remembered where bone marrow is—in the middle of your bone, right next to a ton of nerves.

"Let's get started," Anne said.

As I lay on my stomach, Anne took a scalpel and made a tiny incision in the small of my back. You know how when you cut yourself shaving, you don't feel it right away? Same thing. That wasn't so bad, I thought. But that's because we hadn't really started yet.

How do they harvest bone marrow, you ask?

Good question, one I wish I'd thought to ask. Turns out, it's with a hollow, stainless steel rod about as thick and long as an unsharpened pencil. I glanced at Anne's slight frame and wondered if she had the strength to push what looked like a ten-penny nail through bone. Anne took the rod, slipped it through the hole she'd made in my skin and pushed down until I heard crunching sounds as it penetrated my hip. At first, it just felt like pressure as she ground through the outer part. Not a wonderful feeling but not too bad.

And then she hit the nerve endings.

Try to remember the last time you did something that hurt like hell. Stubbing your toe, maybe. You can remember the incident, but it's hard to remember the pain itself. That's your mind's defense mechanism at work. Our minds don't allow us to remember the true severity of pain, because if you did, it would drive you crazy.

Same thing here.

I remember that it hurt as much as any bone that I've ever broken, but I'm hard pressed to remember the specifics of it. I did what I always do when faced with severe trauma—instead of tightening up, I went completely limp and settled into the pain.

Somehow that made it bearable.

I was careful not to flinch, partly because I was afraid that might cause more pain, and partly because I was showing off for the ladies.

"How's the patient doing?" Anne asked.

"Good," Deborah replied. "I think he just fell asleep."

I mumbled something about how I wasn't asleep, but that I was doing fine and then added, as a joke, "Are we there yet?"

It turned out, we were. Anne had finally arrived at the marrow. She pulled out the instrument, checked it, and then said something I really didn't want to hear.

"We didn't get the sample we needed."

I tried to keep from groaning. "Does this mean you need to create another hole?" I asked.

"No," she said. "Same hole. We just have to go in deeper, that's all."

Oh, boy. Still face down on the table, I gave her the thumbs up to go ahead, and she did. I have no idea how long it took—pain-time is different from real-time—but eventually she got the marrow she needed.

"We'll send it off to the lab," she said, "and I'll let you know as soon as I hear."

She put on a compression bandage and told me I couldn't shower or sweat for twenty-four hours. That sounded like hell to me. I was okay about not sweating for twenty-four hours, but not taking a shower? I don't know about you, but I love my showers. If I'd known that I couldn't take one for a full day, I probably wouldn't have said yes to the whole deal to begin with.

The next day, when the time limit was up, I was finally able to take my shower, followed by a large dinner and a shot of scotch, which helped me fall asleep because it was still daylight out—part of my training plan.

At 2 a.m., the alarm woke me.

I pushed my dogs, Sophia Loren and Stella DuBois, out of bed and let them out to go to the bathroom. They weren't happy because they knew what this meant—I was going to be gone all day on an eighteen-hour bike ride. That's forever in dog time.

An hour later, I was out in the cool night air pedaling my bike down Valley Circle Boulevard in Calabasas. It was fifty-nine degrees outside and I was sweating and shivering. That's normal for a nighttime ride. Ten hours later, in the hundred degree heat of the day, I was still sweating and shivering. That's not normal. But I didn't think anything was really wrong, because I figured that any-one who could ride a bike as long as that couldn't possibly have a problem.

By the middle of the afternoon, my cell phone started ringing.

This was unusual, because anyone who had that number knew not to call me on my big Saturday rides. I ignored the call. But the person called again. And again. And kept calling until I finally had to answer.

It was Deborah. "Hi sweetie," she said. "I know you're on your bike—"

"Yeah," I interrupted, grumpy.

"Get off immediately and take a cab to my house."

"What the hell?" I said. "I'm in the middle of nowhere."

Her voice quavered. "Do not ride another inch. Get a cab to my house as soon as possible."

Everything about this was wrong. Deborah's voice quavering? She was a tough broad, she never quavered. Calling me on a Saturday in the middle of my big ride? Telling me not to go another inch? I knew something was up, but Deborah was prone to exag-geration and, for my sake, I was really hoping she was exaggerating.

I turned around and biked the many miles back to my car.

As soon as I got to the Calabasas Commons, I grabbed myself a large iced coffee at the Starbucks, then drove to Deborah's. When I arrived, I was faced with a dilemma. I hadn't finished my coffee yet, but I didn't think I should bring it in because I didn't want to hear Deborah yelling at me for stopping to get a coffee after I'd promised to get to her place as quickly as possible. While I was debating what to do, I noticed my best friend Andy's car in the driveway.

For the first time during this entire ordeal, I got nervous. What the hell was Andy doing there?

When I walked in, Deborah gave me a big hug. I glanced at Andy. He was stone-faced, pale. This was not going to be good news. I felt like I needed to break the tension.

"No matter what happens here," I said, staring at Andy, "you're still gay, Jewish and balding."

"And you're still an asshole," he replied.

What a relief, I thought. Andy would never tell a dying man he's an asshole!

I was wrong.

Deborah sat me on the couch. "I just want you to know that what I'm about to tell you is, possibly, curable."

I could see in her eyes that she'd rehearsed ten ways of breaking this to me, but I couldn't wait for all that.

"Just give it to me straight," I said.

"You have leukemia."

Chapter Eighteen
I CAN DO BETTER THAN DANIEL DAY LEWIS

WE HAD THE largest graduating class my high school had ever seen, just under one hundred kids. We were together through every year of school, from first grade through twelfth. Of those hundred kids, five of them died before graduation. That's a huge number. To put it in perspective, my dad's graduating class had no deaths, even twenty years after graduation.

The first to die was a girl named Anne. She rode her trike into the street and got hit by a car. She was in the first grade.

The next two were named Ella and Amy. It was seventh grade and they were driving to a friend's house to pick up hand-me-down cheerleader outfits after finding out they were going to be on the cheerleading squad the following year. They were very excited when the Mac truck hit them head on.

The fourth was a guy named Charles. He went duck hunting. While at the lake, he brained a beaver with the butt end of his shotgun. It went off and blew a hole through his chest. He died instantly.

Louise was the fifth one. The police discovered her in her car after it had drifted off the road and into a ditch. She wasn't drunk or speeding or even a bad driver. She'd had an aneurysm. I was one of the few people to see her in the hospital during the twenty-four hours they kept her on life support. I held her hand.

Later, at her funeral in the tiny bayou town of Belle Rose, Louisana, I wept as they put her in the ground. And, standing there in the rain, I realized something. All of us know our birthday but none of us knows our death day. Youth doesn't protect you. Good health doesn't stop it from coming. So I decided, right then, that I wasn't going to be afraid of death. We can't control it, so why be fearful of it?

And that's how I live my life. I rock climb, I ride motorcycles. Can these things kill you? Sure. But something's gonna kill you, so why live in fear?

So, after Deborah told me I had leukemia, my reaction to it was this: a giant sense of relief. Now I knew how it was going to end. The monster was in the room and I could see it.

It also explained a lot of things I'd been wondering about. There were the phantom pains I'd been experiencing. The year before, I was in Big Sky, Montana skiing with Deborah. In the middle of the night, I doubled over in pain with what felt like a knife in my stomach. I would have thrown up if I could have, but only bile came out. It lasted until the afternoon of the next day and then went away without a trace. Over the next year, it happened two more times, finally prompting me to go to a gastroenterologist. After knocking me out and putting a scope down my throat, it turned out that they couldn't find a thing wrong.

Then there were what I called "bicycle comas."

It felt like I had the flu, but without the fever. Usually I would follow up my long ride on Saturday with another long ride on Sunday. But when I was in the grip of one of these "bicycle comas"

I literally couldn't get out of bed. At the time I just thought I was getting older. Who rides a bike that long anyway?

And then there was the weight loss.

I'm 5'11". At my leanest, I weigh a hundred and sixty-five pounds. But during that period, I was down to around one-fifty and that was in spite of eating everything I could get my hands on. Again, my rationale was that I was getting older, maybe even riding too much.

On top of all that, there was the fact that I was shivering all the time. Not to mention that I'd lost my sexual drive, which, for an Italian, is like losing a limb. Believe it or not, in spite of all that, it never even occurred to me that there might be something truly wrong with me. In retrospect it seems so obvious but, as an athlete, I was used to enduring all kinds of strange body issues and behavior.

I know, I know. Earlier, I told you that, when any of my clients complain of an ailment, I'm quick to cancel their workout to protect their health, so why wouldn't I do the same for myself? I think you know why. Do what I say, not what I do. We treat others better than we treat ourselves.

But even though I'd been doing my best to ignore all those weird problems, I still wondered why they were happening. Finally, all those unexplained pains and body issues had an explanation.

Leukemia.

Deborah went on to tell me that I had a rare form we might be able to knock into remission. The problem was that I had so much cancer in me—my bone marrow was about 80 percent leukemia—that they didn't know if my system could survive the amount of chemo it would take to get it into remission. And, as oddly relaxed as I was about hearing the leukemia diagnosis, it was the opposite of how I reacted when I heard the word chemo.

Back in the seventies, my grandmother on my mom's side, Tina Giardina, was diagnosed with breast cancer. They treated it by pouring tons of chemo into her. Over the next couple months, I saw her waste away. At the end, she looked like the Crypt Keeper. She was in terrible pain, both from the cancer and the chemo. There was no life left in her eyes. I was so angry. They'd pumped her full of poison, which left her weak and sick, and she died anyway.

So when I heard the word chemo, all I could picture was suffering through the treatment and then dying anyway. But that wasn't even the worst of it. I'm ashamed to admit it but, when my grandma was dying, I couldn't stand to be around her. Mostly because of the smell. She smelled like death. And I realized that if I had the chemo and wasted away like she did, I wouldn't want anyone to be around me at the end. I couldn't stand the thought of anyone having to endure the smell.

And that was going to be very lonely.

So all of this was going through my mind, but I was sitting there in front of Deborah and Andy and I didn't want to let on how I was really feeling, because real men don't eat quiche or show emotion. So when Deborah said that I was going to have to get on the chemo right away, I told her, "Well, there's only one thing we can do. Throw a chemo party."

Later that night, Deborah and I arrived at an Italian restaurant called Mulholland Grill, where we met a few of my closest friends. The restaurant only served wine, so I made sure we brought our own tequila and scotch.

It was, after all, a party.

Now, I'm not above playing practical jokes and, after I told my friends my diagnosis, I could see that they were hoping this was one of them. But, as the night wore on, and Deborah explained the course of treatment I was about to follow, I could see the truth dawn in all of their eyes.

This was no joke. My leukemia was real.

They stared at me like they were looking at a dead man. I don't blame them. They'd only just found out and weren't sure how to handle it. Hell, I'd only just found out. I was still in shock.

The night ended with each of them hugging and kissing me as they left. When they were gone, I drove down Mulholland and, for the first time, a wave of emotion hit me as I realized that we're all on this planet alone. Even though my friends pledged their love and support—and I was sure they meant it—I realized that none of them could help me get better. I was on my own.

It was a sobering thought.

I spent the better part of the next day trying to figure out how I was going to break the news to my family without getting them too concerned. They were going to want to fly out immediately to help but, if they did, I knew I would feel like I had to entertain them and I didn't want that obligation. I had a lot on my mind. So I told them that the type of leukemia I had was no big deal, the "common cold" of cancer.

As expected, my mom wanted to hop on a plane right away, but I struck a deal with her. I told her if she stayed in Louisiana, I would promise to let her know if things turned bad so that she could come be with me. Reluctantly, she agreed. But now I was going to have to keep the true seriousness of my condition away from my entire family, because I knew they would all talk to each other and I didn't want my mom to get on that plane.

I spent the next two days explaining to each of my clients that this was going to be their last session for a while. When I told them why, most people couldn't believe it. Everyone tried to help in their own way. My Hollywood big-shot clients offered to put me in touch with the best doctors. Others wanted to know if I needed to get off my feet and sit down. Some offered to write checks to hold me over, which I appreciated but never accepted. Some even cried, which really surprised me.

I've been a personal trainer for twenty-five years and, quite honestly, I never thought anyone really cared all that much about me. Like I said, I always thought of myself as the help. I come in, do my thing and then go away. But, almost to a person, everyone's reaction was surprising and touching.

Then there was Dean, my writing partner on this book. He wanted to figure out who was going to play me in the movie based on my life after I was dead.

"Daniel Day Lewis," he said. "He looks kind of like you and he's a great actor."

"Nah," I replied. "I think I can do better."

Dean seemed shocked. "Better than Daniel Day Lewis? He's great looking. He's an Oscar winner!"

I shrugged. "Let's not settle. Let's think about it." We were both trying to ignore the PICC line that was inserted into my arm, giving the hospital a place to attach the chemo pump. "I know who should play you, though," I said.

Dean brightened. "Yeah, who?"

"Paul Giamatti."

He stared at me. "Paul Giamatti? You reject Daniel Day Lewis and I get stuck with Paul Giamatti? Are you crazy!"

"Of course I am. But are we talking about my mental state or trying to cast this movie?"

We never did resolve the argument … although I still think I can do better than Daniel Day Lewis.

The next day, I went to the hospital to begin my chemo treatment.

Cedars-Sinai is an ugly two-tower factory for treating sick people. Deborah and I arrived on a Wednesday morning in her overpriced European sedan. We gave the car to the valet. It's Los Angeles, so even hospitals have valets. I was dreading the admissions process. It always takes forever. There's usually multiple lines and lots of waiting.

What I didn't realize was that I was in the presence of a rock star.

As one of the top radio oncologists in Beverly Hills, Deborah sashayed through Cedars like the headliner at a high-end New Orleans strip joint. All eyes were on her. Usually, checking into a hospital involves lots of little hassles. Your insurance card isn't right. Your name is spelled wrong on a form. You can be delayed for hours.

Not with Deborah.

Every time something like that came up, she gave the person a *look*. Problem solved. In fact, I heard this sentence a lot from the people she dealt with: "We'll take care of it." Within minutes, they put a plastic hospital band around my wrist and led me into the chemo ward.

That's where the star treatment ended.

The light was dim, almost dingy. A fluorescent green. They were probably trying to avoid harsh hospital lighting, but it had the effect of making the sick people there look even sicker. The patients sat in what looked like La-Z-Boy recliners arranged in semi-circles—there had to be over twenty. Maybe as many as forty. It was like a garden of sick people. Next to each recliner was a metal stand that held the chemo for the person in the chair.

From what I could tell, people got their chemo in two different ways.

One was a port in their chest that could be capped between sessions. I found out later that it was for people getting chemo multiple times. It gave the nurses easy access. The other type was for people like me who had PICC lines inserted for a steady supply. But what really struck me was the smell. It reminded me of the smell of my grandmother as she was dying. The smell of death.

This was not something Deborah could fix with a look.

I wanted to turn around and leave. Many of the people in those chairs were bald or wearing scarves on their head. None of them had eyebrows. That's a detail that the movies always seem to get wrong. I think I know why. Eyebrows give people expression, make us look human. Take them away and something suddenly seems off about the person, alien. I doubt actors like to look that way.

The faces around me were pale, with sunken cheekbones. Drawn. It was quiet in there. Library quiet. Whenever someone spoke, you noticed. In the distance, I could see several private rooms with beds. Those were for the truly sick people, the ones who couldn't even sit in a chair.

Deborah led me to a nurse, who started explaining what was going to happen. She held up a machine about the size of a paperback novel.

"This is the pump that's going to administer the chemo," she said.

She pulled out a plastic canister about the size of a thermos in a school lunchbox. There was a bag inside it.

"This is the drug that's going to be administered," she continued. "Now please pay attention, because this can be very dangerous. If this drug leaks out, we need to know right away. Do not touch it with your bare hands. And don't let anyone else touch it. It is not to be touched, understand?"

I said I did. She asked me to sign a piece of paper confirming that.

My God, I thought. They're about to start pumping a drug into my body that can't even be touched by human hands? What am I getting myself into?

Then, almost as an afterthought, the nurse gave me a mini hazmat kit that I could use to safely clean up a spill if one occurred. I grew up near the Gulf Coast of Louisiana and there's one thing you learn when you live there—if a hazmat team is called in, there's a real problem.

But there was a small silver lining. My chemo needed to be administered over the course of a week, which required a hospital stay. Luckily, they agreed to allow me to receive it at Deborah's house, because she was a doctor.

The nurse plugged the medicine into the machine, strapped the machine around my waist, like a fanny pack, and then connected it to the PICC line in my arm. The chemo made a slight sipping sound as it went up the tube. As soon as the line was full of liquid, it began to flow into my veins.

Well, I thought, at least I don't feel nauseous yet.

Soon, we were back in Deborah's car, navigating the choked L.A. streets as we returned to her place. Nestled in the hills of Beverly Hills, Deborah's ranch house was modest in comparison to the mansions next door in Bel Air. My truck was there. My dogs were there. It was going to be my home for the next three weeks.

We went inside. I sat on her couch, staring at her blank television screen and, for the first time in twenty-five years, I realized that there was nothing that had to get done.

It was a strange feeling. I felt like a heavyweight title fight was about to start and I was the arena. The chemo was fighting the cancer in my body while I just sat there, waiting for the outcome. My only job was to keep breathing. I figured that the next month was going to be lonely and quiet as the chemo did its work.

I was wrong.

Chapter Nineteen
SEX, DRUGS AND
ROCK AND ROLL

AS SOON AS my friends heard I was on chemo, I discovered that many of them were pot smokers. And even the dumbest ones, people who'd barely graduated high school, instantly became amateur chemists and botanists.

"Now this strain," one of them might say, "this is Sativa. It has high levels of THC, the active hallucinogen in cannabis which counteracts nausea and the other negative effects of chemo."

"Really?" I'd reply. "Don't you still live with your grandmother?"

Here's something you should know about me. I've never used illicit drugs. Ever. I know that's hard to believe, playing major college football where that stuff is all over the place and sometimes free for players—not to mention living in Los Angeles, dealing with highly creative types who put cocaine on their cornflakes. In spite of being around them all the time, I've never been a drug guy.

Which is why I was stunned at how many people brought me pot as a gift.

Often, it was wrapped very nicely and presented with care. Even my friends who knew I didn't smoke pot still brought me some, along with instructions on how to bake it into cookies and brownies. One woman actually brought me a vaporizer to "make the active ingredient" go down easier.

I took it all with a smile and a thank you. I'm a Southern guy. I was raised to think it's impolite to turn down a gift. And, the truth is, if I'd gotten really nauseated, I probably would have smoked some of it. I hate feeling nauseated so much it actually makes me sick to my stomach. But I never needed to touch the stuff, because the hospital gave me some pills called Kytril to relieve the nausea. They worked well enough that I never had to resort to the pot.

Months later, I wasn't sure what to do with my newfound stash, so I threw it all in a bag and took it to a friend of mine in Hermosa Beach. I knew she was a pot smoker and figured maybe I'd get laid in the process.

We're being honest, right?

So she opened the bag, saw what was inside and started laughing.

"What's so funny?" I asked.

"You have over a pound of pot in here! If you'd gotten pulled over, they'd have nailed you for felony possession with intent to sell."

Not only are my pot-smoking friends amateur chemists, they're also amateur lawyers.

By the way, about getting laid that night ... yeah, that happened.

And, during that period, it happened a lot more than I would have imagined. I don't know if it was charity or if women thought their vaginas had magical healing powers, but I had a surprising number of opportunities while I was hooked up to that chemo pump in Deborah's house.

And I accepted them. Who wouldn't?

Here's how it started. This girl—who I'd modeled with a few years back—came to see me after a particularly rough day. I'd slept most of it in what I thought of as a "chemo coma." It was late at night and she was on her way home from a dinner party. She thought I might be up because I slept at odd hours. It turned out she was right. We visited, had a nice time, but I got tired again. I got tired a lot then.

I offered to let her sleep on the couch while I went into the bedroom and she gratefully accepted. An hour or so later, I woke up and passed her on the way to the bathroom. She was still up. One thing led to another and, for the first time in as long as I could remember, I found myself having sex. Now, you have to understand, I'd lost my sex drive half-a-year earlier which, for me, was like losing my will to live.

Turns out that the cancer had robbed me of testosterone, which had a couple unexpected side effects. My hair, which had been thinning, started getting thicker. Not bad. But I also found myself weeping in movies. Unfortunately, I'm not talking about *Old Yeller*, the only movie a guy's allowed to weep in. I'm talking about girl movies. And what was I even doing in girl movies? Hell, I found myself choked up during commercials for the ASPCA and women's feminine products.

Even though I had parted with my sex drive, suddenly, it came back. Not all the way. Just a little. But a little was enough. So we bumped uglies.

And it was comedy.

The chemo pump was strapped to my waist, which made things … awkward. I tried to move it to the side, but it was still in the way. While I was juggling that, I was also trying to protect the tubing from getting ripped out of the PICC line in my arm. If that happened, it would have sprayed chemo everywhere, causing me to have to bust open the hazmat kit to clean us off like seagulls after the Valdez spill.

That would have been hard to explain.

But as crazy as the situation was, it was fun and, for the first time in a while, I felt alive. After all, can't have sex when you're dead. I couldn't even remember the last time I'd had sex and now I started to wonder if this was going to be the last time. Who knew if I was even going to survive another day? Erections were a rare occurrence, like a solar eclipse or a basketball player that's never been arrested, and I had to make each one count.

I did my best.

Now, what really made all this crazy was that the hospital had warned me about being careful to avoid getting sick. I wasn't supposed to touch anyone. They even gave me anti-bacterial soap. There was a long list of instructions, all designed to keep me free from germs so that my weakened immune system wouldn't get further compromised. It probably never even occurred to them to mention, "Oh, and also don't have sex." Mostly, I'm guessing, because they never thought anyone in their right mind would be interested in doing that.

I began to lose track of time.

The chemo lasted eight days, but I remained at Deborah's for another two and a half weeks because, even though the chemo was finished, it was still in my body, working away at the cancer. The doctors told me that this was when I would feel the most miserable, and they weren't lying. A lot of that was because of the Neupogen, a drug I had to take to boost my white blood cell count.

The nurses said that the Neupogen made your bones feel broken. They were right. My hips felt like they'd been shattered. No matter how I moved, the pain wouldn't go away. Not only was it painful, it was fifteen hundred dollars a shot, money I didn't have. I needed one shot a day. Luckily, insurance covered it. The hospital also gave me a prescription for Vicodin and Oxycontin to help with the pain, but I never filled those prescriptions. Pride, I guess. I thought I could gut my way through it.

I underestimated how tough it would be.

One night, I was alone in the house, nauseated, feeling like crap. Every bone in my body felt broken. I felt like I was two hundred years old. My pee was rust colored. It was like that all the time during the chemo but I noticed it even more on this day. That was the only time I thought, game over. This is it.

That was my lowest point.

And I didn't even have any Vicodin to ease the pain. I thought about smoking some of the pot, but I wasn't sure if pot helped with pain and I also wasn't sure how you went about smoking it. Finally, I remembered that Deborah had a nice bar in her house, so I poured myself a glass of scotch and hoped that would help.

Even though I was feeling like crap, feeling sorry for myself, deep down I knew it wasn't over for me. It wasn't my time to die. I had unfinished business. Things that needed doing. I'm sure that most people have exciting things on their bucket list. Jumping out of airplanes, climbing Mt. Kilimanjaro, a romantic week in Rome. My bucket list, on the other hand, ended up filled with weird shit.

On it, in no particular order:

I wanted to go to Alaska. Mostly because I've been to every other state, along with many countries around the world, but for some reason I'd never been there. The completist in me wanted to check it out.

I wanted to own a Ferrari. Like I said, I'm not a money guy, but damn those Ferraris are nice looking, don't you think? Or maybe they just look that way through my Italian eyes.

I wanted to know if I'd ever been in love. To be clear, I wasn't wishing to fall in love, although that would have been okay if it happened. I mostly wanted to know if I'd ever really been in love, because I wasn't sure. Hell, I couldn't even understand why most people would like me, much less love me, much less have me love them back.

But, most of all, I wanted to finish the Furnace Creek 508. It seems crazy, but if Ahab had his white whale, I had the 508.

And that's what I was thinking about as I waited to see if the chemo had done its job, leaving me cancer free. Or if it had failed, leaving me even sicker than before.

I wouldn't know the answer to that for six long weeks.

* * *

"Vinnie, right?"

I stared at the girl behind the reception desk at Dr. Anne's office, wondering how in the world she knew my name. It had been over two months since I'd been there. Did she have some sort of photographic memory and just knew the names of all the patients she met?

I glanced around at the people in the waiting room and noticed how old they were. Did she know me because I was one of the younger guys there? As I tried to figure it out, the receptionist turned to one of the other women behind the counter and said, "By the way, that's the John Wayne that doesn't need anesthesia for a bone marrow biopsy."

The other woman looked up at me, curious. "That's *the* Vinnie?"

I don't know if I'm *the* Vinnie, I thought. I'm sure there're other Vinnie's.

Hearing my name, Dr. Anne leaned out of her office and gave me a little wave. "Hey, Vinnie!"

I walked over to her and smiled. "What a warm reception I'm getting around here."

"Oh, you have no idea. You've become a real celebrity in the office. Everyone knows the story of the guy who did a bone marrow biopsy with no anesthesia."

I laughed pleasantly but inside I was dying a little because I realized what that meant. I was about to have to get another bone marrow biopsy … without anesthesia.

Couldn't disappoint my fans.

Aside from the terrible pain, the procedure went off without a hitch. Anne got the bone marrow she needed and sent it off to the lab.

While I waited for the results, I went back to training my clients. I was optimistic about what I thought the tests would show. Physically, I felt great. Better than I'd felt in a long time. My sex drive had returned and, to top it all off, I only needed eight hours of sleep as opposed to the fifteen I'd required at the height of my sickness. I was certain that when the results came in, I would have a clean bill of health.

Which is why it was such a shock to discover that the leukemia was still there.

"You're showing improvement," Dr. Anne said, looking at my chart. "We've reduced the amount of cancer in your system, but we haven't gotten rid of it completely. We don't know if the remaining leukemia cells are dead ones being flushed out of your body or live ones that the chemo didn't kill."

"So what do we do?" I asked.

"Well, we give it another six weeks and then check again. It's possible that, by then, your body will have flushed the rest of the cancer cells out of your system and you'll be in the clear."

"And if not?"

"Then we need to put you on another round of chemo and start over."

Shit, I thought. But I wasn't upset about not getting a clean bill of health. I was upset about having to get another bone marrow biopsy—the John Wayne way.

Six weeks later, that's exactly what I did. Oddly enough, by then I'd gotten so used to them that I was able to tell Anne when she was deep enough in the bone to strike marrow.

"You're not there yet," I said while she was grinding through my hip with the steel tube.

"You can tell?" Anne replied in disbelief.

"Yeah. There's a different kind of pain when you're on the marrow."

I'd become a connoisseur of pain.

Anne turned to her assistant. "We never get feedback like that, do we?"

"Nope," the assistant said with a shake of her head. "But that's probably because everyone else is unconscious."

So Anne took the marrow sample and, once again, the waiting game began. Three days later, I got a phone call. It was Anne.

"You're cancer free," she said in the same tone a mechanic might use to let you know your car is ready. "You can resume your normal life."

"Resume your normal life" was a good way to put it because one of the hardest things about the whole ordeal was how abnormal my life had become. I wasn't used to being so passive, to sitting back and watching while my destiny was determined by something I couldn't control. I thanked Anne for all her help. Her kindness and steadiness had helped make everything much more tolerable.

But it was time to resume my normal life.

Truth be told, I'd already resumed my normal life a few months earlier. I couldn't help myself. I was desperate to get back into training mode, because I was only truly happy when I was active, when I was pushing myself to the limit. That's a phrase I've always detested, by the way, mostly because of that last word.

Limit.

It's so ... limiting.

In the 1968 Summer Olympics, Bob Beamon broke the world long jump record with a jump of 29 feet 2 1/2 inches. Records in that event are usually bettered in increments of half or even quarter inches, but he had nearly jumped an astonishing two feet farther than the previous world record. In fact, he'd jumped past the measuring equipment at the Olympics because, at the time, no one contemplated that a jump of that distance was even possible. People thought that the human body couldn't take such an impact, that an athlete's knees would explode upon landing.

Bob Beamon redefined what everyone always thought of as the limit.

His record wasn't bettered for over twenty years.

Back in the fifties, people thought that running a mile in under four minutes was crazy talk—until Roger Bannister did it in a time of 3 minutes 59.4 seconds. These days, a sub four-minute mile is common.

Roger Bannister redefined the limits.

Up until the late seventies, doctors, scientists and mountaineers were all certain of one thing. Reaching the summit of Mt. Everest without supplemental oxygen was a physical impossibility.

They believed a person at that altitude without bottled air would die from lack of oxygen, that there was a barrier a thousand feet below the summit beyond which humans couldn't survive. That is, until Reinhold Messner did it in 1978. Today, an Everest summit without supplemental oxygen is done on a regular basis. And the only reason that this record will never be broken is because there's no summit on Earth higher than Everest.

Reinhold Messner redefined the limits of what people thought the human body could endure. We have, as a species, done this over and over. Why?

Because we are not weak.

We are strong.

But you wouldn't know it by looking around. The reason? We've become civilized.

Look at our boxers. The best of them have always been immigrants—the poor, the working class. These people had nothing to lose. They were literally fighting for their dinner. They're the ones who had to claw and scrape their way to the top. But, almost to a person, once they achieved fame and money, they lost their edge. Or, as Mick tells Rocky in *Rocky 3*, "Three years ago you were supernatural. You was hard and nasty. You had this cast iron jaw. But then the worst thing happened to you that could happen to any fighter. You got civilized!"

So am I saying getting civilized is bad? Absolutely not. I don't want those e-mails. I got enough coming with this damn book already. I'm just using it as a metaphor to describe what happens to us when things get too easy.

We're not weak. We make ourselves weak.

How?

By eating crap we know will make us fat.

By lying on the couch, watching TV instead of moving.

By telling ourselves and our kids that "everyone is a winner" which makes us complacent and removes our natural drive to succeed.

I'm going to say it again. We are not weak—we've just allowed the world to make us that way.

We are strong.

I want to tell you about the worst client I ever had. This guy was in bad shape. Thin arms, big belly. He was a good thirty-five pounds overweight. Let's call him Dean, because that's his name. He's also my co-author on this book—but this was a while ago.

Dean hired me to help him get into shape. He wanted to drop the weight and put on a little muscle. I did my best. I swear.

But this guy was impossible.

He hated working out more than anyone I have ever known. He did the usual things—cancel appointments, feign illness. And, when he did show up, he would try to get me to bullshit about movies and politics in the hopes that I'd forget to tell him to actually, you know, lift some weights or do a couple jump ropes.

But I was onto him.

I made him do that stuff anyway. What I couldn't make him do was eat right. Not that I didn't try. In fact, I took him on an eye-opening tour through his refrigerator and pantry and told him that even fat Elvis, during the rhinestone-studded onesie years, ate healthier than he did. Dean nodded and agreed and then completely ignored me.

In fact, he won't admit it, but I think he was actually glad when I got cancer, because it meant he didn't have to work out for a while.

But I kept at him.

I decided I was not going to give up on this guy. I was going to get him in shape and get him healthy no matter what it took. I gave it my all.

Which he rewarded by firing me.

Truth be told, I was glad. He'd worn me down. But I was also kind of sad because I really liked hanging out with the guy. I figured I'd never see him again, which is why it was such a surprise when he called me the following week and asked if I wanted to grab dinner and drink some beers at King's Fish House. Not only had he given up on getting into shape, he was trying to drag me down with him. But I missed the bald bastard so I showed up.

We became friends.

I didn't want to lose the friendship by urging him into fitness, but after a while I noticed that he started to lose a little weight. I mentioned it, but didn't push it any further. Then I noticed him keeping an eye on what I ordered at dinner—usually a piece of fish and some vegetables. He started to do the same. I told him about No Sugar, No Grains.

The weight kept dropping off.

Eventually, there came a day when he asked, very casually, if there were any exercises he might consider doing, "You know, easy ones that don't take much effort."

Sure, I told him. How about walking? Everyone can do that. It's easy and fun.

He started walking, short distances at first. Then, over time, he'd add on a mile here and there. He told me he was enjoying it. He would have just kept taking his long walks but, one day, he realized he was going to be late for a meeting, so he jogged the rest of the way home.

And he liked it.

So he started jogging a little more. I complimented him on his continued weight loss and improved fitness. He thanked me and then asked another question, again very casually.

"How would I go about putting on some muscle without any pain or effort?"

Everything with this guy required "no pain or effort."

I shrugged and told him about the handful of exercises that give you the most bang for your buck—the ones I told you about in a previous chapter. In fact, I even showed him how to do them.

He nodded, said thanks and didn't mention it again.

Over the next few months, I began to see some results on him and I suggested, very nonchalantly, that, since he was running so much now, he might consider running a 10K or a half-marathon, which is just over thirteen miles. The Malibu Marathon was coming up in a couple months. Why not give it a shot?

He said no. He thought it sounded too difficult.

"Isn't there some kind of training program you need to go through first to be able to do something like that?" he asked.

I shook my head. "Those programs were created for people trying to get faster. You just need to run more. I can show you how to do that safely."

So he started running a little more, building up his aerobic base. Eventually, it was the day of the marathon. When he showed up, I realized he didn't have anything in the way of gear. Hell, he didn't even have an appropriate shirt to wear.

I gave him one of mine.

I also asked my girlfriend, Serena, to run along with him to help him keep a steady pace so he didn't burn out. As an avid marathoner, she happily agreed because she could run a half with her eyes closed.

When we got to the race, I was shocked to see how attractive all the runners were. Then I realized we were in Malibu. Figures.

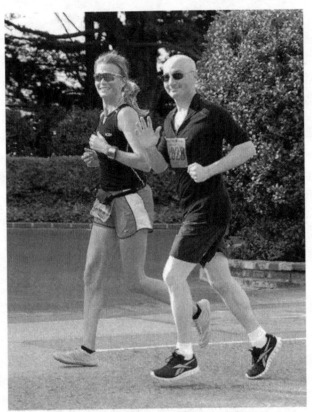

Dean Lorey and Serena Scott Thomas running
the Malibu Half-Marathon.

So the race began. It followed a beautiful route that wound its way along the Pacific coastline. A couple hours later, Dean crossed the finish line, which also marked his crossing over from being a couch potato to being an athlete.

Let's recap what happened here.

He was never an athlete in school. He'd never laced up a pair of running shoes for a 5k or 10k. His job as a TV writer meant that he spent most of his day sitting at a table with a bunch of other writers, trying to avoid the candy jar. He'd started out on this adventure a good thirty pounds overweight and had very little muscle tone. Even worse, he thought of himself as weak.

A few months later, he'd finished a half-marathon with a very respectable time.

If you want to see what he's up to, check him out at www.deanlorey.com. He writes about stuff he worked on, like *Arrested Development* and the *Nightmare Academy* book series, as well as his road to fitness. As I said, Dean was my worst client, and I've had some pretty bad ones, trust me. If he can turn it around, so can you. Hell, so can anyone. So let me say it one more time.

We all face obstacles in life. I faced a big one. But we are not weak.

We are strong.

Part Four

CUT THE CRAP

Chapter Twenty
TIME TO TAKE THE TRASH OUT

I WALKED INTO my local Starbucks and ran into an old buddy of mine, comedian John Mendoza. You'd recognize him. He has a face like a catcher's mitt.

"How's your finger?" he asked.

"It's fine," I said, a little confused.

"You better never lose that thing, 'cause your career would be over."

"Really? Why?"

He smiled. "Because all you do is point."

He demonstrated with a pretty good impression of me. I knew exactly what he was talking about. When I train people, I use a lot of pointing and hand gestures to show them what exercise to do next. Speaking with your hands is an Italian thing. I can only speak one language with my mouth, but my hands are multi-lingual.

Besides, I'm usually in the middle of telling a story that's totally unrelated to fitness and I hate to interrupt myself when I'm talking.

There's a method to that madness. I'll go out of my way to chat about anything other than the task at hand because I want to take my client's minds off the discomfort and repetition of the exercise. Ever see those TV trainers that yell and count and pretend they're drill sergeants?

"Come on, you can do it! Give me five more! Breathe! Feel the buuuuurn!"

What's up with those assholes? You know why they do that? Because they've seen other trainers do it, so they think they should. They're perpetuating a stereotype that should have been put out to pasture along with VCRs, phone booths and Tony Little's pony tail. When you're exercising, you're going to get the same amount of benefit whether you're enjoying yourself or not, so I figure why not make it fun? Or, as I tell my clients:

Your body doesn't mind if your brain's having a good time.

It's like when I go to the dentist. When he's drilling my teeth, there's usually a certain amount of pain involved. You know what he's doing while I'm in pain? He's talking. About anything. The weather, what movies he's seen, sports. Any kind of bullshit he can think of to take my mind off the pain.

You know what he's not doing? Getting in my face and yelling, "Feel the pain, Vinnie! Listen to the sound of my high-speed drill as it cuts into your teeth! Smell your enamel buuuurn!"

Speaking of dentists, while one of my clients was doing bench presses, I told him this story.

"I was talking to my dentist," I said, "and I asked him what's the weirdest thing he ever pulled out of someone's gums. You know what he told me? 'There's never any shortage of pubic hair in there.'"

I'll talk to my clients about anything to make the workout more fun. Far as I'm concerned, absolutely nothing is off limits. Like this little gem I shared with another client of mine.

"I have a third ball," I told him while he was on the elliptical. "You think I'm kidding? I really do. I have three. I hear most guys only have two." Then I went on to explain that it's not technically an authentic testicle—it's really a fibrous growth that appeared after the chemo. "After I discovered it wasn't cancerous," I continued, "a surgeon wanted to remove it but I told the guy, 'Are you kidding? Makes me unique. A third nut may not put me in a class by myself but it can't take that long to call role.'"

There's no reason a workout shouldn't be fun. A good trainer should help make it that way, and the best ones are truly on your side. They're your buddy, your partner in crime. The way you look should be even more important to them than the way they look.

Remember Mick from *Rocky*? He was Rocky's trainer. Mick wasn't winning any beauty pageants. Hell, he'd lose to Mendoza. But Mick cared about Rocky and they were on his journey together. Why is that important?

Because there's strength in numbers.

That's why people join running and cycling clubs. These aren't things you do with a partner. No one can run for you. No one can pedal for you. But people join these organizations because they want support. Because it's more fun. Because there's strength in numbers.

In 1962, JFK gave a speech at Rice University where he talked about the goal of sending a man to the moon. The big question was why. Not only was it going to be expensive, it was going to be incredibly difficult, if not impossible. JFK had an answer. He said that we choose to do these things "not because they are easy, but because they are hard."

That's an elegant way of saying "cut the crap."

We do things that are worthwhile, not because they're easy, but because they're hard. Let me give you an example.

I want to tell you about a client of mine. Caroline. You'd like her. There's a lot of loud-mouthed, New York Italian lady stuffed into her compact four-eleven frame. She's funny. With that accent, if you were talking to her on the phone, you'd swear she was Bugs

Bunny's sister. She uses the F-word as a noun, verb and adjective. She may only weigh a hundred pounds, but ninety of that is heart. She's run over twenty marathons, including Boston, and recently completed the Ironman triathlon—all while holding down a full-time job.

She is, to put it mildly, a badass.

She also has Lupus, an auto-immune disease that causes a person's immune system to attack the healthy tissues in their body. The list of complications from this disease is too long and scary to mention. There is no cure. But, in spite of all that, she works harder than anyone I know. I often see her in the pre-dawn hours on the street, getting her run in.

Caroline cut the crap. She did it not because it was easy, but because it was hard.

What about Amy Dodson? Have you ever heard of her? If not, you should have. She's an elementary school teacher in Arizona who discovered that she loved to run. She began with local 5Ks and 10Ks, then moved up to ten-milers, half-marathons and, finally, marathons.

But she didn't stop there.

Next came the triathlon, where she won two national and two world championships. After that, she completed a couple Ironmans, followed by a 50K race in Toronto, which led to four fifty-mile runs, which qualified her for the Western States 100 Endurance Run, maybe the toughest trail race out there. Just accomplishing all of this, while holding down a full-time job, is an incredible feat. But what if I told you she did it without one of her legs?

And then what if I told you that that wasn't even the tough part.

She also did it with only one lung.

At the age of nineteen, Amy had her left leg amputated and her lung removed to save her from cancer. It worked. I first met her in the scorching July heat of Death Valley where she was pacing a competitor in the one hundred and thirty five mile Badwater race. She was so fun, vivacious and positive that it honestly took me a long time to realize she was missing a leg.

Do me a favor. Google her. See if you can find a picture where she's not smiling.

Amy Dodson cut the crap. She did it not because it was easy, but because it was hard.

Let me ask the question you're probably thinking. Why do people do these crazy things—triathlons, ultra sports where the distances are too insane for most people to comprehend, climbing mountains so high that you have to bring your own oxygen? Is it because they pay well?

Nope.

In fact they cost money. Lots of money, particularly when you're talking about something like a mountain climbing expedition to Nepal, where the price of entry is in the tens of thousands of dollars. Same for RAAM, the Race Across America. Some people say it can be done for twenty thousand. Everyone I know that's done it has spent at least thirty. And that's just for the race. Forget about the cost of training.

So if it doesn't pay well, there must be some other tangible benefit to doing this stuff, right? Does it help you career wise?

Nope.

Just the opposite. Not only does it require a large financial investment, it requires a large time investment. Just training for these things can easily take twenty-five or more hours a week for months on end. Time that could be spent advancing your career.

How about helping in your relationships with friends and family?

Nope.

Hell, I've lost relationships over this sport. Friendships, girlfriends. There are just not enough hours in the day to work, train and also put in the time that relationships require. I can't tell you how many girlfriends have told me, "You're more in love with that bike than me."

It's hard to argue. I do love my bike.

Riding is my passion and I've always looked for someone to share it, not change it. In fact, it wasn't until I met Serena that I found a relationship that worked. She's not even a cyclist, she's a runner—but passion is passion.

It's hard to find someone like that. I got lucky.

I remember, years ago, an eighteen-year old kid came up to me before an ultra cycling race I was competing in. He said he wanted to be an ultra cyclist and asked me how much weight he could lose without sacrificing power. I asked him if he had a girl-friend. He said he did. I asked him how much she weighed.

"About a hundred and twenty," he said.

"That's the first weight you're going to have to lose."

Funny thing is, I really meant it at the time. I guess I was a little cynical back then.

So, if these crazy events don't benefit your finances, career or relationships, why do people do them? I have three answers for you. Here's the first one.

Why do people do these things?

Answer: why not?

Remember what Rocky said after Adrian asked him, "Why do you wanna fight?" He replied, "Because I can't sing or dance."

Look, I don't mean to trivialize the question, but why do you assume people have a choice? Some of us just can't sing or dance. Not only that, I could name a lot of other pursuits that people spend time and money on that don't benefit them financially, career-wise or in their relationships.

Some people love fantasy football. Some people love to col-lect stamps. Some people play video games. You could probably name a hundred more.

None of these things benefit people in a practical way, and yet people do them because they like to. Because they can't sing or dance. Because it's the key that fits their particular lock. The truth is, you'll never know if it's your key until you try it. Who knows? It may unlock a door in you that you never even knew could be opened.

So that's the first reason why people enjoy doing these insane events. Here's the second.

The problem with life is that it's not a game.

We love games! Board games, card games, video games. They're fun. They have levels, goals, winners and losers. Many of them even have a finish line. But life has none of those things, except maybe a finish line but the finish line is death and that's no fun.

Hell, the Scientologists even created a religion around turning life into a game, a science-fiction one, with levels and fancy sci-fi equipment and even space aliens you have to defeat. I think they're nuts but what do I know? A lot of people seem to like them. They even own an entire town in Florida and I'm still working on getting a couch.

Point is, even though we know life isn't a game, we try to make it one. We give ourselves arbitrary goals to get momentary satisfaction. A better car, a raise, a nicer house. The problem with all those things is that your happiness is tied to something unworthy. Money. In fact, that's how I decide whether or not to buy something. I try to put a dollar price on the happiness. If I look at a new computer that costs a thousand bucks, I think to myself, will it make me a thousand bucks happier?

If the answer is "no," and it usually is, I pass.

So that's the second reason people love these kinds of events. They put clear rules, goals and objectives over something as muddy as life. They give us a way to win that relies on our own ability, determination and willpower.

But there's one more reason I love these competitions, even though they don't help you financially, career-wise or in your relationships.

I don't love them in spite of those things.

I love them because of those things.

Taking the money out of the equation keeps it pure. It's just you and the sport.

As far as career goes, I guess it does have some impact on my career but I've never gained a client because I competed in ultras, although I've gained them because of the special knowledge my personal experience brings.

And, as for relationships, the truth is I don't want a relationship with someone who doesn't understand this passion. It separates the wheat from the chaff.

It may sound crazy, but it's like in *Rocky 3* when Mick asks Rocky, "Does anything normal go through your head?" and Rocky answers, "Nothing that I remember." What's weird to the other guy is normal to me. And maybe it's normal for you, too, and you just don't know it yet.

Who knows, maybe you can't sing or dance either.

But Vinnie, you're probably thinking, what you're asking is impossible. If cutting the crap means I have to run an ironman competition or become some kind of ultra runner, forget it! There's no way I'm ever going to be able to do that stuff!

I understand your hesitation, but first I'd like to remind you that Caroline finished an Ironman triathlon with lupus and Amy became a national and world champion while missing about a half a body. They did it. You want to tell me again that you can't?

Truth is, I'm not even asking you to do what they did, although I'd love it if you gave it a shot, because this isn't about amazing accomplishments. It's about the everyday accomplishments. It's about doing something not because it's easy, but because it's hard.

When I started riding a bike through New Orleans instead of using a car ... that was me cutting the crap.

When I bought the bike with pizza money and forced myself to start eating better food ... that was me cutting the crap.

The first time you pass on a jelly doughnut or take the stairs instead of the elevator or sign up for a local dance class, that's you cutting the crap. And you should give yourself credit. All those books and videos out there want to make money by selling you on the idea that you can get the body you want with no effort, that you can get something for nothing.

You know what that does?

It makes you quit in frustration because you don't see the results they promise. And if you do stick with it and start seeing results, it makes your hard work seem like nothing. It minimizes your accomplishment, because these things are not easy. They are hard. But when you do them, that's you cutting the crap. Being out there every day, trying your best—that's the most important thing. And you know what's going to happen when you do that?

You're going to fail.

Look, everyone cares about IQ but I care about FQ—Failure Quotient. Failure is good. Failure is necessary. Failure means you're in the game! If you've never failed, you've never played. Look at it this way. Times are tough out there right now and a lot of people are looking for work. Chances are, you're going to go on a lot of job interviews and you're going to hear "no" a lot. Doesn't matter. You only need to hear one "yes."

Want to know how many times I've failed?

I'd need another book just to skim the surface, but I'll tell you about one time in particular. Remember that actress I told you about in the opening of the book, the one where her people promised to pay me ten grand if I could take thirty-five pounds off her? I did it. It turned out that the actress was so heavy that the thirty-five pounds flew off.

She was thrilled, as you might imagine. I knew the Hollywood types were going to be thrilled, as well. Which is why it was such a shock when her managers and the studio called me back into the conference room.

"You did a wonderful job," they said. "Her body looks great. But we have a problem."

They all glanced at each other nervously. No one wanted to be the one to say what this problem was. Must be a hell of a problem, I thought.

Finally, they laid their cards on the table. "It's her face. Can you make her lose more weight in her face?"

I stared at them. Had I heard right? "She just has a round face," I said, finally. "That's just the way her face is."

They all looked away. Suddenly, their shoes and the ceiling became the most interesting things on the planet. "Right," they continued. "We completely understand."

Good, I thought. Finally.

"But can you get her to lose some weight in her face?" they pressed. "In the screen test, it's still coming off too fat."

I felt like I was in a Fellini film. So, futilely, I tried to explain to them how weight loss works, that you can't just lose weight in a particular area. I also explained that you can't change a person's basic biology. You can't make a short guy tall just by working out. They nodded and didn't care. They wanted more weight to come off.

The actress and I had worked hard and done everything they wanted us to do and it still wasn't enough for these Hollywood types.

By the time her show was cancelled, she'd gained all the weight back.

Why? Because she was doing it for all the wrong reasons ... and so was I. I wanted to look like a hero and save the day, not to mention make some bucks, so I went against my principles and got her weight off quickly. But I taught her nothing. She did what I asked her to do, but I didn't give her any knowledge or resources. I didn't support her.

I consider that whole episode a failure.

But I learned something. It's not enough to help people. You have to show them how to help themselves because you won't always be there. Even more important, for fitness to work long term, the client has to want it for the right reasons.

Look at Dean, my co-author. I worked out with him for months and he barely improved because he wasn't ready. He didn't want it. It wasn't until years later, when he returned to working out, that he finally saw big results. Nothing had changed. He was still the same guy, but the difference was that he wanted it then. He was ready.

The problem right now is that not enough people are ready. When I look at the world today, I see the same thing happening to fitness that's happening to the economy. In fact, I call it:

The economy of fitness.

Just like we've lost the economic middle class in the country, we've lost the middle class of fit people. We're left with only couch potatoes and ultra athletes. It wasn't always that way. Back in the sixties, only 13 percent of Americans were considered obese. By 2005, that increased to 35 percent. And that's just obesity. If you look at the statistics for Americans who are currently at a weight that's considered "unhealthy," the number skyrockets to over two thirds of the country.

Two thirds. That's the middle class that we've lost. I want to bring them back.

How? Simple. Stay away from sugars and grains. Exercise. Cut the crap.

At the beginning of this thing, I told you that I was your personal trainer and I am. There's strength in numbers. With you and me, that's two. That's a good start. But it's just that, a start. Join a gym, a cycling club, a hiking group. Find other people out there looking to do the same thing. You see all those old people walking around malls in the morning before the stores open? Go walk with them. They could use some company.

And don't let the bad stuff that everyone else is eating throw you off your game. Next time you go out to a restaurant and they bring some bread to the table, cut the crap! Tell them to take it away. You don't eat it at home before dinner so why should you eat it when you go out?

And don't let those bums selling worthless fitness gear and useless supplements con you into wasting your hard earned cash. Tell them to go screw themselves. Tell them to cut the crap.

And next time you see a celebrity on TV telling you to try Jenny or Weight Watchers or any of the other pre-packaged diet-food factories, keep in mind you've already tried them. You hated them then and you're going to hate them now.

I want to tell you one more story before we go.

You know who Joe Dean is? He's one of the greatest men that ever lived. He started off as the sales director for Converse tennis shoes, then he became the athletic director for LSU and turned the sports program into what it is today. More importantly, he was a mentor to me when I was a teenager. He had many stories, but this was the one that's gotten me through life so far.

"Vinnie," he said, "you ever go to throw away a soda can, and when you open the trash you see it's full, so you try to teeter the can on top and close the lid so it's someone else's problem?"

"Sure, Mr. Dean," I told him. "I've done that."

"Next time you see that," he said, "I want you to do something completely different. Don't wait for your parents to tell you to empty it. Take the initiative and do it yourself." He ended by saying, "In life, whenever the trash can is full, don't wait for someone else to deal with it. Just take it out."

We've been neglecting ourselves for too long. For most of our lives, we've delayed getting the kind of healthy body and active life we want and deserve.

The trash can is now full, folks.

Let's take it out.

LAGNIAPPE

Book's over. You can stop reading right now and tell your friends you finished and no one would call you a liar. But, like I said a while back, I'm from Louisiana and we have this thing called lagniappe, meaning a little something extra, which is what I'm going to give you right now.

Before I knew if my cancer was in remission, I'd started training again. My thinking was that if the leukemia was gone, then I'd already have a solid jump on preparing for the Furnace Creek 508. But if I wasn't in remission, then I figured it couldn't hurt to get into better physical and mental shape before my next round of chemo. Either way, I didn't see any reason not to train.

So, by the time I got the all clear from the doctor, I didn't have the heart to tell her that I'd already laid down three thousand miles on the bike. My aerobic base was solid. The problem was that, between the chemo and the cancer, I'd lost a ton of muscle mass. Plus, I didn't have an ounce of fat on me and I was going to need some in order to fuel my body during the intense training ahead.

This put me in a bizarre position.

Usually, I'm helping people lose fat, not put it on, so I became a living example of "do what I say, not what I do." I started eating at least a pint of Ben and Jerry's a night (Chunky Monkey was a favorite) along with tons of pasta. Sugar and grains pack on those pounds, right?

Because I wasn't used to the intense sugar spikes that were always followed by a crash, I started dumping heavy cream onto my Chunky Monkey. I know what you're thinking, that's like taking sand to the beach. But here's why it helped. Fat, which heavy cream is full of, slows your body's absorption of carbs, which helps prevent those terrible spikes.

Over the next six months, I trained relentlessly.

By September, I had logged over twelve thousand miles on the bike. As for putting on muscle and fat, it was a struggle. My body was so depleted by the end of the chemo that I couldn't overcome the massive amount of calories I was burning during training. I wasn't concerned about this, because I was still foolishly using sugar and grains as my primary fuel. Old habits die hard. The food I ate during the race was going to have to get me to the finish line, but because I wasn't yet following a "No Sugar/No Grains" lifestyle, I hoped it would be enough.

This turned out to be a critical error ... but I would only learn that during the race. The hard way.

The race began in the parking lot of the Hilton Garden Inn in Santa Clarita, a nice but modest hotel surrounded by California palms. It shared a parking lot with a Marie Calendar's restaurant and was within walking distance of Six Flags Magic Mountain theme park. In other words, if you were in the mood for a slice of pie or a roller coaster ride, this was the place to be. But pie and roller coasters were not on my mind.

Failure was.

The other racers waited at the starting line under the hotel's overhang, listening to Chris Kostman, the race director, as he gave final instructions. When he was done, he played the National Anthem on a boombox, amplified by his bullhorn.

I was nowhere near there.

I was back in the parking lot by my rented, white Toyota van, joking with my crew, trying to take my mind off things. I didn't want to be buried in the pack, waiting for the race to start. The nervous energy of other competitors was infectious and I had plenty of nerves already without any help from them.

Not only had I DNFd (Did Not Finish) the last time I'd run this race, there was something else weighing on my mind. Something even worse. A couple months earlier, as a test to see if my body could handle this kind of distance, I'd competed in the Race Across Oregon, or RAO. It's a five hundred thirty-five mile trek through the mountains of Oregon with forty thousand feet of elevation gain. It's grueling. Not as tough as the Furnace Creek 508, with its ripping wind, dry desert heat and freezing night-time cold, but it's close.

I'd hoped to have a strong finish in the RAO to give me confidence heading into the 508, but I ended up DNFing after four hundred miles. The problem was my stomach. After only a hundred miles it began to bother me. Have you ever had too much to eat and felt that, if you ate even one more bite, you'd puke? That's the way this felt, but I didn't have anything in my stomach. I grew so nauseated that I couldn't even keep down water. I tried drinking some Pellegrino ("Italian water for an Italian stomach!") because, in the past, the bubbles had helped soothe my nausea, but not even that worked.

At the three-hundred-thirty mile mark, an EMT team visited me on the course and determined that I was severely dehydrated and should quit the race and get immediate medical attention. I refused, against their advice and the wishes of my crew, preferring to push on and try to finish. I literally willed my body to the four-hundred mile mark, but by then, I was in serious trouble.

I was so dehydrated that my muscles were seizing. The spasms were agonizing. I'd also become disoriented and could no longer even pedal in a straight line. My crew, consisting of Mehran (my crew chief from my prior 508 attempt), David Holt (a veteran of the sport who I'd crewed for at a previous 508) and my new girl-friend, Serena (who I was hoping to impress), finally said "no more." I had no fight left in me to argue. I was done.

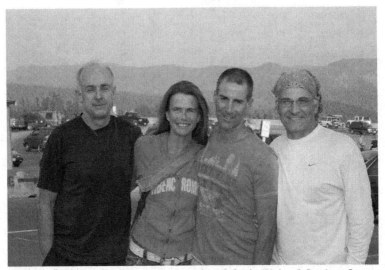

Me with David Holt, Serena Scott Thomas and Mehran Salamati before the 500 plus mile Race Across Oregon.

The Race Across Oregon was supposed to give me confidence for the Furnace Creek 508, but instead, I had DNFd and in spectacular fashion.

That's what I was thinking about as I waited for the 508 to begin. Would my stomach hold up? What about my knee, the one that had crapped out on me the last time I was here? I was also coming off two DNFs in a row. I wasn't used to failure, but failure was becoming my norm. My body was the one thing I could always count on, even when other things were bad. It had always been strong. But after the leukemia and the chemo, my confidence was shaken.

Over the loudspeaker, I heard Chris Kostman begin the countdown to the start of the race. "Ten ... nine ... eight ..."

I mounted my bike and pedaled over to the pack.

"seven ... six ... five ... four ..."

Calm down, I told myself. Just relax. Cut the crap.

"three ... two ... one!"

I took a breath and pushed down on my pedal as all the competitors surged forward.

FIRST STAGE
SANTA CLARITA TO CALIFORNIA CITY
(Mile 0–82.25 / Elevation Gain: 6,176')

WE LEFT THE parking lot accompanied by a police escort. The cops formed a moving line in front of the racers, clearing the path and holding everyone to a comfortable fifteen mile an hour speed, like pace cars at a NASCAR race. This is called a neutral start, part of the pageantry of the sport, but also necessary to get us safely out of town. The police escorted us five miles, holding traffic, blocking lights, until we got out onto open road.

I glanced around at the other cyclists. It was like looking in a mirror. They all had lean, sinewy bodies, oversized quads, undersized calves, faces gaunt. Their lack of fat made even the younger competitors look older than they were. In fact, the average age of the competitors is usually a shock to most people when they first experience an ultra like this. They expect to see a group of twenty-somethings, because who else would have the strength and stamina to handle forty-plus hours of straight riding? The truth is that it's not uncommon for fifty-year-olds to win the thing outright, which has happened several times. Remember, David Holt, my crew chief, came in second on a previous race and he was nearing sixty.

The whole notion that athletics are for the young is turned upside down in ultra sports, where youthful competitors are often left scratching their heads as people twice their age sail past. It's not about young legs, it's about wisdom and experience. As my wise Italian friend, Enzo Valentino, puts it, "An old chicken makes a good broth." Or, as I always say:

> *It's not about how fast you can go long,*
> *it's about how long you can go fast.*

Once we cleared the town, the cops peeled away and the road became like Pamplona during the running of the bulls. Filled with pent-up nervous energy, the competitors exploded forward. I was toward the middle front of the pack, hoping to avoid the jumble that often occurs at the back. With the town behind us, we began to spread out as we made our way through country roads in the chill morning air. The fog was heavy and I could only see as far as the person in front of me. It was like riding through soup.

In spite of the cold temperature and limited visibility, I was feeling great, passing people as I began the climb to where we would eventually meet up with our crew vans for the first time. This was considered the unsupported part of the race, meaning we were cut off from our support vehicles until mile twenty-nine.

It was freezing cold and drizzling at the top of Johnson Road where I finally met my van. As I approached, I could see the words "Pound Puppy" written on a hand-lettered sign taped to the back. That was my totem. For reasons unbeknownst to anyone, Chris Kostman decided that, instead of using numbers to identify racers, like every other race on planet Earth, we would be identified by animals, otherwise known as our "totems."

I picked Pound Puppy because I love dogs and, during my previous 508, I was raising money for the Lange Foundation, a charity that rescues dogs and cats that would otherwise be destroyed in pounds. This year, my charity was Maximum Hope, a cancer foundation founded by actor Brad Garret, but my totem was still Pound Puppy. Once you've established the name for your totem, you have it for life.

As I sped past the van, David, my crew chief, shouted, "Slow down! You're going out too fast! You're gonna blow up!"

"Blow up" is an ultra term for starting too hard and then fizzling out before the end, resulting in a DNF.

I knew he was right, but the only thing I cared about at that point was speeding down the mountain to a lower altitude where I knew it would be warmer. I hate the cold. I shiver. I shake. I'm a warm weather guy and I was determined to get warm, fast. So I got myself into an aerodynamic tuck with my face just inches above the handlebars, and flew down the mountain at more than fifty-miles-an-hour, feeling great. Ten minutes later, I was at the foot of the Mojave desert, where the air was dry and the temperature was a sunny eighty degrees.

I was off to a good start.

Soon, I found myself biking through the desert surrounded by hundreds of giant, white windmills in what is known as the Windmill Climb. My favorite. In a sport not known for people with climbing ability, I climb well. There are plenty of racers out there who can take me on the flats, but I'm tough to beat on a climb. In fact, whenever I pass someone going uphill, I usually shout, "See you when you pass me back on the flats!"

And they often do.

I was feeling strong. My left knee, the reason I had DNFd on the previous 508, was solid and my stomach was as quiet as nap-time in a preschool. As I sped past the town of Mojave, I was near the head of the pack, in second or third place. Oddly, I didn't care if I was high up in the standings. I was just hoping to finish and I didn't want the pressure of being chased for the next thirty hours, so I was waiting for people to start passing me.

Soon, I arrived at the first checkpoint in California City.

Let's talk about California City. I've been to plenty of cities named after the state they're in. Kansas City comes to mind. Nice place. You can go shopping, hit a bar. You need a night on the town? Kansas City can deliver. They even have a pro-football team, not to mention that you can get a great steak. Let's compare that to California City. Can you get a great steak? Sure, no problem! As long as you catch the cow, butcher it and cook it yourself.

There's nothing in California City.

I sped past the first checkpoint, which was manned by a couple volunteer race officials sitting on folding chairs, while my crew stopped to check me in. I had completed the first stage with a great time and I was in great spirits. I was off to a terrific start.

STAGE TWO
CALIFORNIA CITY TO TRONA
(Mile 82.25–152.5 / Total Elevation Gain: 10,388')

I'D ALREADY BEEN pedaling for over eighty miles by the time Stage Two began. Most avid cyclists aspire to reach the century mark, which is a hundred miles. That's about the length of four marathons, a hell of a good distance. In fact, a hundred miles is usually the finish line on charity rides, but in the world of ultra cycling, a hundred miles is just a warm up. Even though we'd been racing for several hours, we were just getting started.

As I rode through the flats, I kept expecting other cyclists to pass me, but that didn't happen because I was reaping the benefit of a strong tail wind that helped compensate for what was usually the weakest part of my race. My crew van, following the strict race rules for daylight hours, hop-scotched ahead of me and continued down the road until pulling over to wait for me to pass.

As I sped by, I grabbed the water bottle Serena held out for me. I continued down the road, sipping at it, while Serena noted the time and amount of water I'd received on my race log. The crew kept meticulous records of my food and water intake because they were in charge of making sure that I stayed hydrated and consumed at least two-hundred and fifty calories per hour, which is all the stomach can process in that amount of time.

Serena hopped back into the van with the rest of the crew, where they watched until I disappeared from sight. I was thrilled to have her on my team. She had prior crewing experience and her dry British humor was great at keeping everyone's morale up. Besides, who wouldn't want Dr. Molly Warmflash from *The World Is Not Enough* handing them water in the desert?

As much as I loved my crew, I was disappointed that my good buddy Mehran, who had been my crew chief during my last several races, couldn't make it. His father was ill and he needed to be at the man's side. Luckily, David was available to take his place. I was glad about this for two reasons. First, as an ultra athlete himself, he's a great addition to any crew. But, more importantly, I figured if he was sitting in my van, he couldn't be on the course, kicking my ass.

Still feeling great and with the wind at my back, I sailed past the second checkpoint at Trona.

Remember how California City was a wasteland? It's Paris compared to Trona. In fact, as each rider and crew passed through, they momentarily doubled the town's population. My van pulled over to check me in and refuel, while I pushed on to Stage Three.

STAGE THREE
TRONA TO FURNACE CREEK
(Mile 152.5–251.7 / Total Elevation Gain: 17,926')

FURNACE CREEK IS the midway point of the entire race but, to get there, you have to endure the Pass.

Townes Pass.

It doesn't look like much from the flats—a gentle climb that disappears into a mountain—but that easy stretch soon turns into an agonizing 13 percent slope. Whether you reach it during the day or in the dark of night, you know you're on it. And you're on it for a long time. It seems to take forever, plus a week. Even though it's thirteen miles from base to summit, that only tells part of the story.

The climb to get there is over a vertical mile.

To put that in perspective, imagine climbing up the Empire State Building. Now imagine climbing up three and a half Empire State Buildings in a row. That's how high a vertical mile is. Now imagine doing it after you've been hammering away on your bike for over two hundred miles, which is how far you've gone when you arrive at the foot of the Pass. The climb is so grueling, in fact, that some competitors simply get off their bikes and walk during the toughest parts.

I was one of the first competitors to arrive at the Pass, having benefited from that powerful tailwind for the last hundred miles. It was still daytime, which was a good sign, and my legs felt strong considering the constant pedaling I'd been doing for the last nine-and-a-half hours. But as soon as I made the turn to begin the climb, which almost paradoxically faces you in the opposite direction, that tailwind turned against me.

It was like hitting a wall. Not gale force, but enough to knock my speed down from the over twenty-miles-an-hour I'd been enjoying to less than half that. In fact, I was going so slowly that, as I passed my crew van, we had enough time to exchange a couple sentences.

"Do you need anything?" Serena yelled.

"Steroids!" I shouted back, laughing. Then, "No, I just need to be on my own."

She knew what that meant, that I needed some space to get into a rhythm. But for the next forty-five minutes, I couldn't do it. I was used to fighting steep grades during my training but not with this kind of wind. I could feel my legs filling with lactic acid and, as soon as they started burning, I'd rise into a standing position and pedal a few strokes to let the acid drain out and stop them from cooking. No matter what I did, I couldn't find a comfortable position.

And that wasn't the worst of it.

For the first time during the race, my stomach began acting up. It wasn't too bad, just a mild discomfort, but I knew that it could get out of hand, fast, and I didn't want a repeat of the Race Across Oregon. I became focused on reaching the summit, hoping that my stomach troubles would go away once I was on the downhill. But getting there wasn't going to be easy.

Between the steep grade and the wind, I felt like I was in a wind tunnel. At one point, my speed slowed to a turtle-like four-miles-an-hour. I was going so slow, in fact, that David got out of the van and walked alongside me for a stretch.

"How you feeling?" he asked.

"I need Pellegrino," I said between breaths.

"Shit, how bad is it?"

David knew that asking for Pellegrino meant I was having stomach problems. Carbonated drinks can settle an upset stomach, so asking for one is like a neon sign that says, "I'm in trouble." In fact, months earlier while training in Santa Barbara, I was struggling because my stomach was empty and sour. I knew I needed to get some calories and bubbles into it right away, so I walked into a convenience store and bought a beer, which I figured was like liquid bread.

It was, and it worked, although I wouldn't have even considered doing the same thing during the 508, because drinking any sort of alcohol during the race was strictly against the rules.

"How bad is it?" David repeated.

"Not like Oregon," I replied. "But I don't want it to get there."

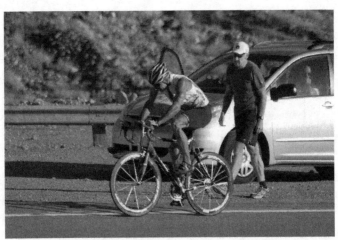

Moving so slowly up Towne Pass that David was able to walk next to me!

He hustled back to the van and sped ahead of me while Serena filled a water bottle with Pellegrino. She handed it off to me as I rode past. I drank it and it helped a little, but I had a feeling that this wasn't going to be the last time I heard from my stomach.

Soon, the steep grade began to flatten out, which told me that I was nearing the summit. I knew I was going to have to make a mandatory stop once I reached the bottom to add lights to my bike while the crew prepared the van for night-time conditions. I hoped that my stomach would settle itself on the downhill ride because I wanted to eat some food during the break, but I could only do that if my stomach was calm.

Once I crested the summit, my speed went from six-miles-an-hour, the pace of a jogger, to twenty, then forty, until finally topping out at just over fifty-five miles per hour. I was flying down the backside of the mountain, hurtling toward the lowest point in the Western hemisphere, Death Valley.

Behind me, the field had spread out. Racers were strewn from the beginning of the Pass all the way back to Trona. They were going to have to fight the mountain at night, in the dark and the cold—something I was happy to avoid.

Finally, I arrived at the bottom of the Pass and saw my van up ahead pulled over on the side of the road. It was getting close to 6 p.m., which meant that lights had to be added to my handlebars and the van had to have yellow flashers installed to give ample warning to approaching traffic. Any deviation could result in instant disqualification.

As I'd hoped, the ride down the Pass settled my stomach a bit and I had a couple minutes to eat before I needed to get back on the road. Serena offered a few options. Slices of mozzarella cheese on a piece of bread, a peanut butter and jelly sandwich, a turkey sandwich, as well as a beef burrito from the taco stand back in Trona—now gone, sadly.

Best tacos in the world.

I had a few bites of the burrito and asked Serena to put the mozzarella sandwich in a baggie. I shoved it into my jersey pocket for later, then got back on the bike and headed into the town of Stovepipe Wells, knowing that I was less than twenty miles from the halfway point, marked by the race's namesake town of Furnace Creek. But that small psychological boost was quickly dashed when the storm hit.

It started with the wind, whipping across the salt flats of Death Valley. I'd been fighting wind all the way up the Pass, but this time it came at me from the side so powerfully that I had to lean my entire body against it just to stay upright. It was like leaning against a wall.

And with the wind came the sand.

It swirled across the desert in thick sheets, stinging my face and cutting visibility. I suddenly felt like I had a good idea what people went through during dermabrasion. The sky up ahead was black. Bolts of lightning flashed, dancing across the desert floor. It was apocalyptic. Biblical. I could see the rain sweeping toward me, darkening the salt flats. And then it was on me—big, heavy drops.

I began to get concerned.

Flash floods were common in the desert and it was no joke to get swept away by one. But then something else grabbed my attention, something that worried me even more. I glanced up to see two rainbows far ahead, one above the other.

Oh, hell, I thought. Am I getting delirious? Am I seeing double? It seemed like too early in the race for that but I had to be sure.

I gestured for the van to drive up alongside me. Even though it wasn't full dark yet, all crew vehicles had to stay "as closely as safety permits" to their rider. We call it the invisible tether.

Serena rolled down the window. "What do you need?"

"You see a rainbow?" I asked, fighting to keep the bike straight as the wind threatened to push me into the van.

Serena nodded. "Yeah."

I hesitated before asking the next question, scared of what the answer might be. "Do you see two rainbows?"

Serena started laughing. She knew exactly what I was worried about. "Yeah, there are two. And they're beautiful."

I smiled to let the van know I was okay. They dropped back behind me as I pressed on.

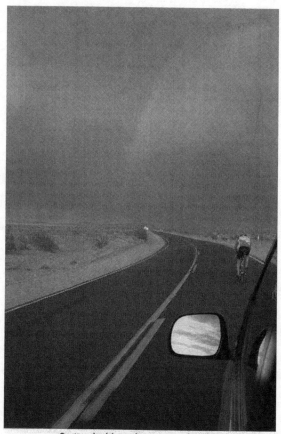

Seeing double rainbows in Death Valley.

Minutes later, the sun set, taking the rainbows with it. The desert was dark except for the little pocket where I rode, illuminated by the van's headlights. Finally, as the storm began to ease, I rolled into the next checkpoint at a lonely gas station in the tiny town of Furnace Creek.

STAGE FOUR
FURNACE CREEK TO SHOSHONE
(Mile 251.7–325.3 / Total Elevation Gain: 24,670')

WHILE THE CREW checked me in, I ate some of the mozzarella sandwich and then greased the inside of my thighs with chamois cream to help prevent chafing. Some riders, at this point, like to change into a fresh pair of riding shorts because they think it helps them avoid blisters. My attitude is, if the first pair is working, I'm going to stick with them.

David walked up to me. "You're in seventh place," he said.

He probably thought I'd be upset by that, because earlier I'd been as high up as second, but I didn't care. My only goal was to finish. Besides, seventh place was great. I was just glad to be on what I considered the "right" side of the Pass. Most of the pack were still either on it or dreading the thought of it. Some of them wouldn't get to where I was standing until morning.

I climbed back on my bike and, with the van only a few feet behind me, left the little oasis town of Furnace Creek and headed into the long dark of the desert. For the next couple hours, my stomach felt solid and my legs were strong, considering they were nearing three hundred miles of straight pedaling.

Even though I felt good, it was like riding through a black abyss, which made everything more difficult. Even something as simple as controlling my speed was a challenge because I had no reference points. I could see only the road beneath my wheels, lit by the van behind me. Looking anywhere else was like looking into a dark curtain, featureless and dead.

And then, a breakthrough.

I began to be able to make out shapes. The spindly branches of the Joshua trees, the barrel cactus sticking out of the ground like fat fingers. Even the salt flats were beginning to shimmer. But it wasn't sunrise, that was still hours away. I looked up to see that the storm had passed and the clouds had cleared, revealing a bright, full moon that lit up the desert.

I've always thought of Death Valley as one of the most beautiful places on Earth. It's stark and vast and empty, like the ocean floor it once was. I've often wished that the 508 started in Death Valley, so I could ride through it during the day, but it was almost as spectacular at night. Just seeing it gave me a little boost.

I continued making my way through its alien landscape until the road swept left to reveal the foot of Jubilee Pass, the first of two climbs that provided our escape route out of the deep bowl of Death Valley. It rose over fifteen hundred feet above the desert floor.

I started up, followed closely by the van. I was doing okay until, suddenly, I felt the first pangs of the thing I dreaded most.

My stomach started to shut down.

It's like this. When you're racing for an extreme length of time, you get most of your fuel from the food you put into your body. If you stop eating, you run out, just like when a car runs out of gas. But even though I was only feeling mildly nauseated, I knew from experience that the feeling would increase ten-fold as soon as I started chewing. Even the concept of food was upsetting my stomach. It became impossible to even think about eating, much less eat, much less keep food down even if I could. But if I couldn't eat, I was going to run out of gas, fast.

And that wasn't the worst of it.

Even more important than eating is staying hydrated. If you fall behind on your calorie intake, you can sometimes fight back after you get some food into your stomach, but there's no fighting back from dehydration. You're done. Game over. It's like trying to put toothpaste back into the tube.

Which is why I had to figure out a way to get some food and liquid into my body during the climb. Because chewing was a guaranteed route to puking, my only shot was to take in liquid nutrition by drinking a product called Pediasure, designed to give sick kids the nutrients they need during their illness. The problem is that it's filled with sugar, which can shut you down on these long races— but I was out of options.

I drank some and it gave me the calorie boost I needed. Unfortunately, the sugar was causing my stomach to feel bloated, which made me feel like throwing up. I needed another plan, and fast. Even though we weren't talking about it, it was hard to escape the fact that this was looking like Race Across Oregon all over again.

I pulled over and we decided that the best course of action was for me to take short breaks, two or three minutes at a stretch, to let my stomach settle enough so that I could try to eat some simple foods that would help soak up the acid and clear the nausea. Saltines, bread, accompanied by some water. This helped, but I knew it wasn't going to be a long-term fix. With close to two-hundred miles left in the race, Band-Aids weren't going to do the trick.

Steve, one of my other crew members, suggested I try an over-the-counter antacid that he happened to have on him. I was reluctant. One of the most basic rules of sporting events is that you never change anything on game day. If you haven't tried it in practice, don't do it during the game. That statement is never truer than in ultra sports. Because of the extremes of time and distance, everything becomes magnified. Even something as simple as trying new shoes or shorts is an almost incomprehensible gamble.

With that in mind, I decided to pass on the antacid. I wanted to try to get to the top of Jubilee climb, followed by the even more severe Salsberry climb, without taking such a huge risk. I figured that once I was out of Death Valley, we could reassess the situation.

Spitting up bile, I gutted my way to the top of Jubilee. After a brief downhill respite, I soldiered up Salsberry, which was almost another two-thousand feet of climbing.

Sometime after midnight, in the early morning hours, I crested the top of Salsberry and, looking down at the flickering yellow dots of the caution lights on the crew vans ahead of me, I began the welcome descent into the town of Shoshone. When I arrived at the checkpoint, I discovered that I had dropped from 7th to 13th place, but at least I was still in the game.

STAGE FIVE
SHOSHONE TO BAKER
(Mile 325.3–381.6 / Total Elevation Gain: 26,856')

3 A.M. DEAD OF night. The sun wasn't coming up until six, which seemed like a year away. Those were the hardest hours, when exhaustion dragged at me like an anchor. Daylight seemed like a dream.

I was able to choke down some food in Shoshone and my stomach had settled a little, but eating was still a problem, as was drinking. In fact, at my pee stops, one of the crew members, usually David, would inspect my urine with a flashlight, studying its color and texture. Brown, foamy piss meant you were dehydrated, which is big time bad. Not to sound like a cheap beer ad, but mine was a nice amber with low foam, just what you want in a urine sample.

Since we're on the subject, these stops took place alongside the road. The desert has a surprising lack of port-a-potties. You do what you have to do. There's no room for modesty in ultra sports. Hell, the daughter of a good friend of mine, while crewing for her dad, had to pee out of the side of the van as it raced down the road. Usually, when I stopped to go to the bathroom, so would the rest of the crew. Serena called it "splashing my boots."

It sounds better when you hear it in a British accent.

The biggest problem during these long, dark hours was the terrible need to sleep. I'd been awake nearly one full day. It began to feel like torture, like I was a prisoner of war and they were trying to break me down.

At times, I would be pedaling and suddenly hear the van's horn and realize that I'd actually fallen asleep on the bike. My eyes would snap open and I'd see that I had nearly veered off the asphalt or into the oncoming lane. I sometimes tried to stay awake by aiming my bike toward the reflective lane dividers (otherwise known as "drunk bumps") in the middle of the road. The jarring helped keep me awake but, as I grew more tired, they became blurry and then doubled in my vision and I had trouble even seeing them to hit them.

And falling asleep wasn't just a problem for the riders. The crew struggled as well. They had been awake as long as I had and the monotony of following a cyclist, hour after endless hour, took its toll. Even though they took turns driving and napping, I still found myself nervous about them falling asleep at the wheel and running me down.

They were, after all, only ten feet behind.

Even though my stomach had settled a little, I still hadn't eaten anywhere near enough calories and I was running on fumes. We tried to do a "sleep reset" where I pulled over, got into the van and slept for five minutes before being loudly shaken awake by the crew and hurried back onto my bike. In the past, this technique had helped reset my body's internal clock, leaving me awake and refreshed, at least somewhat. But, after two tries, I realized it wasn't working. Not only that, my stomach was growing worse by the minute.

It was time for drastic measures. If things didn't change quickly, I knew I wouldn't be able to keep my eyes open or swallow any food or drink and the race would be over. Out of desperation, I decided to try two things.

First, I agreed to take some antacid to settle my stomach, even though trying an untested medication during a race went against the most fundamental rule followed by ultra athletes everywhere.

Second, I agreed to take a twenty-minute nap in the van, which meant that I would wake at sunup. The hope was that the small amount of sleep, followed by daylight, would finally reset my body's internal clock.

With serious reservations but seeing no alternative, I took the antacid, climbed into the van and went to sleep. During the thirty minutes I was unconscious, David and the rest of the crew watched in despair as other cyclists ambled past, putting me farther and farther behind.

Thirty minutes later, I woke to find that my stomach was, amazingly, calm and, although still exhausted, I felt like I could keep my eyes open. I began riding again.

It was day two.

With the morning sun warming my face, I pedaled the ten miles to my next checkpoint in Baker. I was hurting bad, but compared to what I had been feeling, bad was an improvement. As I rode, I belched several times which opened up my stomach, releasing the bloat. Things were moving around down there again and, for the first time since Trona, I experienced a welcome feeling.

Hunger. I was starving.

Up ahead, I could see what's billed as "the world's biggest thermometer" rising into the air above the town of Baker. It would be hot by afternoon but, at dawn, it was still cool and pleasant. The thermometer wasn't my destination, however, world's biggest or not. I needed to eat and there was only one game in town.

The Mad Greek.

STAGE SIX
BAKER TO KELSO
(Mile 381.6–416.5 / Total Elevation Gain: 29,776')

I THINK I know what the Mad Greek is so mad about.

He must have woken up one morning, hung over from ouzo, and said to himself, "Why the hell did I build a Greek restaurant out in the middle of the desert?" Because of its proximity to Vegas, the only explanation for the existence of the Mad Greek is that the poor son of a bitch who owns it lost a bet. The faded sign on top promises "something for everybody," and it's not lying, as long as the "something" you want is a gyro, and the "everybody" who wants it has no problem eating in an outdoor dining area that looks like the love child of McDonald's and the Parthenon.

I rolled up to the mini-me statue of David in the parking lot, leaned my bike against his junk, then walked inside and up to the clerk where I mumbled, "Double cheeseburger and a shake. Don't worry, somebody will pay you, okay?"

He stared at my salt-crusted, gaunt face and nodded.

I shuffled to the nearest booth, dropped in and waited. Within minutes, Serena entered, clearly concerned. I could see she thought I'd given up.

"How are you doing?" she asked.

"Pretty beat up."

"You want to take your shoes off for a minute?"

I shook my head. "I'm scared if I take them off, my feet will swell and I'll never get them back on. Go take care of yourself. Get some food. I got some coming."

She kissed me on the cheek, licked the salt from her lips and, smiling, said, "You taste like a potato chip." Then she headed to the counter as David and Steve walked in the front door. Steve, being a rookie and not quite knowing what to say, busied himself by heading to the bathroom while David came over to me.

"You good?" he asked.

I nodded. "I'm gonna finish."

He smiled. "That's what I wanted to hear. You know you still have another twenty-four hours to do this thing. We're all prepared to stay another night if we have to."

"How's Serena holding up?" I asked.

He shrugged. "She hates to see you in pain."

I knew what he was talking about because I often crewed for him with his wife, Susan, during his races. There was no shortage of tears when things got rough, and they always did.

"You know, David," I said, "we won't need the whole twenty-four hours. I'll get us to the finish before sunset."

"That's a good goal to have," he replied. "It's just not a bad idea to have a back-up plan."

"We won't need one. I've got demons chasing me. I gotta finish. This ain't Race Across Oregon. I'm not leaving this course alive."

He stared at me a long time.

Just then, my double cheeseburger showed up, along with a strawberry shake that had a straw and umbrella in it. Adorable. We both looked at each other and started laughing. I picked up the burger and took a bite. It was so damn good I made it disappear faster than an eight-ball at Charlie Sheen's house. It was maybe the best thing I'd ever tasted.

And don't even get me started on the shake …

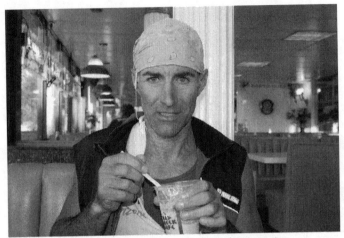

The meal that saved the day at the Mad Greek, Death Valley, Ca.

After we'd all eaten, I went outside and pulled my bike off the statue of David. What was an Italian statue doing outside a Greek diner, anyway? Then I pedaled back onto the course. Daytime rules meant the van didn't have to be tethered to me any more, so they left me on my own while they refueled.

The climb out of Baker was twenty-two miles and, although it wasn't steep, it was long and I knew it was going to be tough to do on tired legs. But there was some good news. I'd finally been able to hydrate and replenish my calories.

The road to Kelso, which rose a hundred feet every mile, was made interminably worse by the fact that it took place on one of the crappiest roads in America. If there was an award for cracked asphalt, this at least deserved honorable mention. Any part of my body that didn't already hurt started hurting now. Every fiber of my being ached.

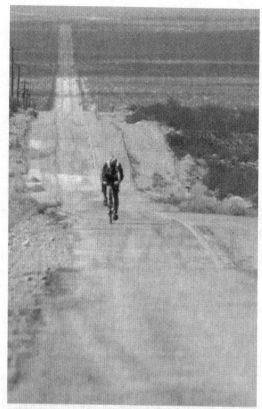

Nineteen competitors in front and seventy behind. In ultras, you always seem to be alone with your thoughts.

As I gutted my way up that endless hill, I found myself flashing back to my time in the chemo ward at Cedars. The nurses who'd put in my PICC line. The other patients sitting in their recliners, faces gray and gaunt, hooked up to their IV's. Hairless. How many of them were still there, getting their treatments, I wondered.

How many of them were still alive?

Truth is I didn't get to know any of those people. Even so, they were still with me and, somehow, they spurred me on. I remembered my grandmother retching in her bed, agonized. There was no way the nausea I had suffered the previous night could come close to equaling what she went through. And yet, there on that long hill, I found myself pulling strength from her pain. From all of their pains.

Me finishing this race wasn't going to miraculously make any of them better. Truth is, I wasn't doing it for them. I was doing it for myself, to prove that I could. I'd been lucky to survive the cancer, that's all. Even though my finishing the race wasn't going to help them, I felt like I had to at least honor them by trying to do my absolute best with the break I'd been given.

Soon, the twenty-two mile climb was behind me and I found myself racing down the backside into Kelso.

Stage six was complete. Only two more stages left to go. That meant nothing, of course. As every racer knows, it ain't over until you're in the house.

STAGE SEVEN
KELSO TO AMBOY
(Mile 416.5–450.3 / Total Elevation Gain: 32,056')

IF THE ROAD to Kelso deserved honorable mention for crappiest road in America, the road to Amboy would win the thing hands down. Deep cracks, loose stones in the roadway like IEDs, it was a vicious spider web of broken concrete slabs held together by crumbling asphalt. The road felt like it was specifically designed to rattle every bone in my body and beat my crotch black and blue while threatening to push the bike seat into my esophagus through my ass. And that's if I could even stay on the damn thing.

I kept my head down and ground on the pedals, hammering away at them like I hated them. My quadriceps screamed in agony. I was in so much pain that I only had two choices. Give up or get pissed.

I got pissed.

It was late in the race, but instead of keeping slow and steady, I pushed myself like a maniac even though the finish line was still hours away. I remembered this road from 2005 when I was crewing for David. It was rough then and that was when I was riding in a van that had full suspension on forgiving radial tires.

Now, I was on a carbon fiber bike with no suspension, riding on tires as hard as the asphalt they rolled over.

I beat that bike like a rented mule, trying like hell to ignore the terrible pounding my body was taking. The lower part of my back on my left side started to hurt. I'm guessing it was my spleen letting me know that it wasn't having a good time. I tried to take my mind off it by concentrating on all the other pains. The ones in my knees, which felt full of broken glass. My swollen, blistered feet. Soon, I noticed a metallic taste in my mouth. It was familiar, but not coppery, like blood. Something else, something even harder to place ...

Chemo.

I realized it was the phantom taste of the chemo that had been coursing through my body. I wanted to believe that I'd sweated it out months ago, but there it was, a shadow of its former self, to remind me of what I'd been through. I kept on, pounding away at the pedals until finally, miraculously, I ended up in the town of Amboy.

Legend has it that the whole, crappy town has been for sale for years. Never had a buyer. No one wants it. That's pretty much all you need to know about Amboy. Truth is I've never been happier to see any place in my entire life, because it meant that Stage Seven was finally over.

Stage Eight—the final stage—was all that stood between me and the finish line.

FINAL STAGE
AMBOY TO TWENTY NINE PALMS
(Mile 450.3–509.5 / Total Elevation Gain: 36,226')

AS I PASSED the last checkpoint and headed toward Twenty-Nine Palms, which was still almost sixty miles away, there was only one thing on my mind.

Toilet paper.

No, I didn't have to go to the bathroom. After each competitor crossed the finish line, the race officials would string up a new piece of toilet paper for the next person to break through.

Seems trivial, right?

But, to me, that piece of toilet paper represented, not the five-hundred miles I rode to get to it, but the twelve-thousand miles of training just to take a shot at it. It represented all the Saturdays I had to wake up, bleary eyed, at 2 a.m. to ride until 2 a.m. the following morning. It represented all the dinners and concerts and movies with friends that I had to miss to keep up my schedule. It represented months of bone-tired exhaustion, of swollen feet, sore necks and calloused hands. It represented the sacrifice of Serena, who I'd started dating in the middle of this, and her willingness to put up with my mistress, the bike. It represented the loyalty of my crew and their selflessness as they gave up their weekend and time with their families to help me on my mad endeavor. Most of all, it represented becoming strong again, being alive.

I know that sounds corny, but so do a lot of true things.

"You're in twentieth place," David had said to me all the way back at the checkpoint in Baker. As soon as he'd said it, I knew what I had to do. Finish no worse than twentieth. I figured that if no one ever passed me, it meant I was still moving forward and if I kept moving forward, eventually I was going to cross the finish line.

As I made my way up Sheephole Summit, a climb only made tough due to the fatigue caused by the four-hundred-and-seventy miles that came before it, I began to get nervous. Even though the finish line wasn't in sight, it was within my grasp, and the sport was littered with stories of riders cramping up, crashing out or collapsing from pure exhaustion just a few short miles from the end.

That wasn't going to happen to me.

As much as my body screamed "stop!" my mind screamed "you will not DNF!" I'd told David that I had demons chasing me across the desert and I did, but they came in funny shapes.

Those horrible nuns from my childhood were there, telling me I was a failure, mocking the way I spoke, saying get the grits out of your mouth.

The kids in my elementary school were there, beating me up, taunting me by calling me "Vinna."

My cancer was there, telling me that my body had turned on me, that it wasn't what it used to be, that it could come back at any time and take me out whenever it wanted to.

But, mostly, the seductive voice of my own self-doubt was there, telling me that there was no need to do this to myself, that it was pointless, that I was a loser, that it would be better for everyone if I just called it a day.

Then I realized that I was the luckiest man on Earth because I was getting another shot. How could I be a loser? I beat fucking cancer. Not only that, I was getting a chance to do something hardly anyone gets to do—redeem myself by trying again. Most people, including me, get lost in the grind of daily life and plan to do the things they really want to do "someday."

But, for me, someday was today.

Over the years, I've had clients who wanted to set me up in business or asked me to come work at their companies for tons of money. They thought I was wasting my life as a trainer. But I didn't think I was wasting my life. I valued what I was doing. I didn't take the money route. I took this route.

And I was going to see it to the end.

I crested the top of Sheephole Summit and enjoyed the breeze on my face as I shot down the other side. At the bottom, I took a right-hand turn and found myself facing the sleepy desert town of Twenty-Nine Palms. The only thing that stood between me and the finish line was forty miles of asphalt. Unfortunately, most of those forty miles were uphill and into the wind.

I kept pedaling.

As I did, I thought about Jack LaLanne who, all those years ago in Bayou Lafourche, spoke volumes to me through a television set. I wasn't paying attention to what he was saying, but what he was doing. He showed me, a kid that felt completely hopeless, that you couldn't control the world but you could control you.

And I thought about Joe Bonadona, the first guy that ever treated me with respect. A man who taught me more about life than fitness and, trust me, he taught me a lot about fitness. I even thought about his cinderblock gym and how hot it got in there. Was it possible that Joe's no-frills, gut-through-it regimen was helping me all these years later?

Yeah, I figured. It was.

And then, there in the distance, halfway up a hill, I saw something I'd been dying to see for what seemed like years. Its real name was the Best Western Gardens Hotel but, as far as I was concerned, it was the summit of Everest, the gold medal ceremony of the 1980 U.S. Men's Olympic hockey team, and the finals at Wimbledon all rolled into one. Most of the year it was just a crappy motel in the desert, but that day it was the finish line of the 2008 Furnace Creek 508.

Exhausted, covered in sweat, salt and sand, with swollen hands and feet, I sailed into the parking lot in front of the hotel where the race officially ended, only to find that they didn't even have a makeshift toilet paper finish line waiting for me.

Didn't matter. Something even better was waiting.

My friends.

My crew was there, cheering me on. So were a handful of scattered spectators. And then, to my surprise, I saw my good friend Mehran, who had not been able to crew for me because of his father's illness. As it turned out, his dad had stabilized, so he'd gathered up a handful of my best friends—Jonathan, Steve, Glen and Christina—packed them into his small plane and flew them out to meet me.

I'd finished in twentieth place.

But my final standing didn't matter a lick. Hell, as far as I was concerned, there was more honor in finishing last than first. In fact, one of my friends, Steve Gray, is legendary for always completing the race mere minutes before the deadline. That guy is my hero. I was on the course for thirty-three hours over a single night. I couldn't even imagine adding another night.

Compare that to Steve.

He'd run the race multiple times and, every year, he was on the course for nearly forty-eight hours over two nights. Want to talk about heart, guts and stamina? You can't do it without talking about Steve Gray.

I kissed Serena, took photos with my friends and then headed into my room at the hotel for a nice, cold shower.

Finally, it was finished. Not just the race, everything. The nuns, the bullying, the demons chasing me across the desert.

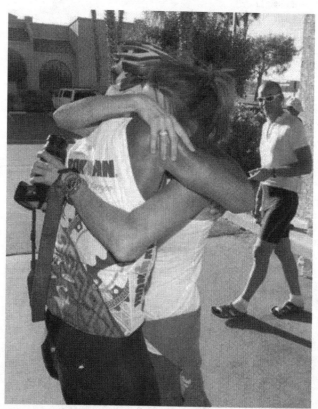

Hugging Serena after crossing the finish line of the Furnace Creek 508. Things get emotional!

Gone. Done. Over.

And so is this book.

I've enjoyed the journey and I hope you have, too. Now I think I might pour myself a glass of scotch—but only one. After all, I have to be up at 4 a.m. I have clients to meet and a training schedule to keep.

Next year's 508 is just around the corner.

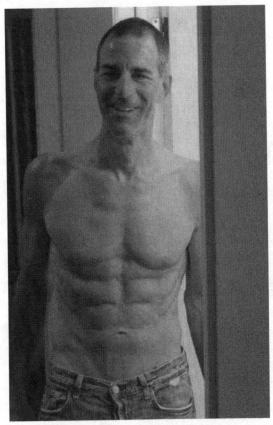

Some racers bloat during ultra races. I emaciate.

ACKNOWLEDGEMENTS

Dean and I faced a dilemma when we sat down to write this book. We hated a lot of the other diet and fitness guides out there, mostly because they took a simple idea and stretched it out to book length. I wanted to help people with something I really believed in, the concept of No Sugar, No Grains. Sure, it requires some explanation ... but a whole book? Boring as hell, right?

After much thought (and watching Shakira videos—she's right, hips really don't lie) we decided to write only as much about No Sugar, No Grains as we felt was essential and entertaining. In other words, we tried to get rid of all the boring stuff and write about everything else. We didn't mind if it was raunchy or painful, as long as it was always true. Anthony Bourdain's *Kitchen Confidential* was an inspiration. We hope you liked it and found it helpful, inspiring, and fun. As you might guess, we didn't do it alone. I have some people I want to thank, and so does Dean.

I want to thank my parents, Marie and Vincent "Cy" Tortorich. As schoolteachers, they taught me that education is everything. My mother, in particular, shared with me her love of books.

I also want to thank Gill Fuller. There comes a time in every-one's life where you have to accept help. She gave it to me when I needed it. I had no way to thank her for everything she did, which is why I'm glad I wrote this book. It gives me a chance to thank her now.

I also want to thank the real ladies behind the fictional names Dr. Deborah and Dr. Anne. Without them, I wouldn't be here to-day. And by "wouldn't be here" I mean "wouldn't be alive." Thank you both.

And, finally, most importantly, I want to thank the love of my life, the woman who can make me laugh and cry, Serena Scott Thomas. Thank you for putting up with me through this whole process. I really couldn't have done any of this without you. I love you, honey.

Dean Lorey here. I just wanted to poke my head in and thank my wife, Elizabeth Lorey. Writing a book is complicated enough, but self-publishing one takes a ton of time and energy. As always, she was terrific throughout. We met over twenty years ago on the set of *Friday the 13th part 9: Jason Goes To Hell* and have been together ever since. I started losing my hair during that movie, but I gained a wonderful wife. I figure that's a pretty good trade. I love you, hun.

About the Authors

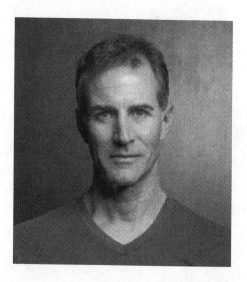

Fitness trainer Vinnie Tortorich has been Hollywood's "go-to" guy for celebrities, athletes and everyday people for over 22 years. After hosting *TALKING FITNESS* (New Orleans' top-rated radio program), he came to Beverly Hills where his guest shot on *THE OPRAH WINFREY SHOW* made it the 7th most watched episode of all time. His *AMERICA'S ANGRIEST TRAINER* podcast reaches hundreds of thousands of listeners, who tune in weekly for his r-rated diet and fitness advice as well as his epic rants.

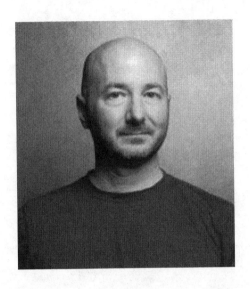

Writer/Producer Dean Lorey was nominated for an Emmy for his work on *ARRESTED DEVELOPMENT*. His film and TV credits include *MAJOR PAYNE, MY WIFE AND KIDS* and many more. His first novel, *NIGHTMARE ACADEMY: MONSTER HUNTERS,* won "Best Children's Novel of the Year, 2008" from the SCIBA. The series is in development at Universal Studios and is published in over 20 countries. Currently, he's an Executive Producer on the upcoming David E. Kelley CBS show *THE CRAZY ONES* starring Robin Williams and Sarah Michelle Gellar.

To stay current with the latest on Vinnie and Dean, you can follow them at their websites.

Vinnie: www.vinnietortorich.com
Dean: www.deanlorey.com

Made in the USA
Lexington, KY
18 November 2018